Sex Tips and Tales from Women Who Dare

I DEDICATE THIS BOOK TO MY PARENTS,

WHO HAVE BEEN A CONSTANT SOURCE OF LOVE

AND SUPPORT IN MY LIFE.

* * *

Ordering

Trade bookstores in the U.S. and Canada, please contact:

Publishers Group West
1700 Fourth Street, Berkeley CA 94710
Phone: (800) 788-3123   Fax: (510) 528-3444

Hunter House books are available at bulk discounts for textbook course adoptions; to qualifying community, health care, and government organizations; and for special promotions and fund-raising. For details please contact:

Special Sales Department
Hunter House Inc., PO Box 2914, Alameda CA 94501-0914
Phone: (510) 865-5282   Fax: (510) 865-4295
E-mail: ordering@hunterhouse.com

Individuals can order our books from most bookstores or by calling toll-free:
(800) 266-5592

Sex Tips & Tales

from Women Who Dare

Exploring the Exotic Erotic

EDITED BY JO-ANNE BAKER

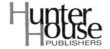

Hunter House PUBLISHERS

Library of Congress Cataloging-in-Publication Data

Baker, Jo-Anne, 1955-
Sex tips and tales from women who dare / edited by Jo-Anne Baker
p. cm.
Includes bibliographical references
ISBN 0-89793-321-4 (pb)
1. Sex instruction for women. 2. Women--Sexual behavior. I. Title.
HQ46 .B217 2001
613.9′6—dc21   2001016616

Project Credits

Cover Design: Jinni Fontana/Kiran Rana/Jil Weil
Book Production: Hunter House
Copy Editor: Kelley Blewster
Proofreader: David Marion
Graphics Coordinator: Ariel Parker
Acquisitions Editor: Jeanne Brondino
Associate Editor: Alexandra Mummery
Editorial and Production Assistant: Melissa Millar
Publicity Manager: Sarah Frederick
Marketing Assistant: Earlita Chenault
Administrator: Theresa Nelson
Customer Service Manager: Christina Sverdrup
Order Fulfillment: Joel Irons
Publisher: Kiran S. Rana

Printed and Bound by Publishers Press, Salt Lake City, Utah

Manufactured in the United States of America
9 8 7 6 5 4 3 2 1   First Edition   01 02 03 04 05

Contents

Acknowledgments

I would like to thank all the women in this book, who have inspired me and given me their words of wisdom and depth of knowledge.

To my mentor and friend Annie Sprinkle, whose generosity of spirit and guidance has made this project possible.

To Kimberly O'Sullivan, for her invaluable help—I would not have been able to compile this book without you.

To Esmé Holmes, for her love and support.

To Ruth Ostrow, who is a wonderful friend and an inspiration.

To my brother Murray Baker, for his sense of humor, kindness, and regular computer support.

To my friend Ron Tanner, who has always steered me in the right direction.

Important Note

The material in this book is intended to provide an overview of sexuality and lifestyle opinions, options, and choices. Every effort has been made to provide accurate and dependable information. However, the activites and exercises described in the book are not prescriptive in any way. Those who wish to try them should make a mature and balanced evaluation of their possible benefits and risks and should look for appropriate professional guidance if they are at all unsure. The author, editors, and publisher cannot be held responsible for any outcomes that derive from a person or persons trying the activities and approaches described in this book, either on their own or under the care of a licensed professional.

Introduction

Women have always been at the forefront of sexual revolution. From the nineteenth century, when feminists fought Victorian moral hypocrisy, to the present day, women have understood the link between personal freedom and freedom of sexual expression. Often these pioneering women are forgotten, yet the names of their male counterparts—Baron von Richard Krafft-Ebing, Freud, and Reich—have been immortalized in the language of sexuality. Few people remember Victoria Woodhull or Sylvia Pankhurst, who spoke out for women's sexual rights and against the social stigmatization of sex workers and of women who wished to celebrate their female eroticism.

By the 1960s women throughout the Western world had been affected by the enormous social changes of the decade. Central to those changes were emphases on the right to individual expression and on many social freedoms, including the right to sexual freedom. With the advent of improved and more effective contraception, particularly the Pill, sex and pregnancy could be separated from each other for the first time in history.

This allowed women to take more sexual risks, to start thinking about their own sexual fulfillment, and to question traditional female roles and the nature of their relationships. However, as women started expressing their need for personal and sexual freedom, they often ran into societal obstacles. Women found, more often than not, that the 1960s and 1970s ideal of an individual's right to love and live as one chose did not apply to them and that strong social stigmas were still attached to women who were sexually free and unashamed of their desire.

The women's movement of the 1970s was a natural extension of this period as women reappraised all aspects of their lives and how they had been taught by society what a woman should be. While there was much debate and discussion about female liberation, the area of sexuality remained problematic. Over the next two decades, sexual rights, responsibilities, lifestyles, and choices were hotly debated. At the same time, some women identified with the archetypes of earth mother and the ancient goddesses and embraced a New Age philosophy of how a woman should live.

The last decade of the twentieth century has seen another sexual revolution, one based on sex positivism, the concept that sex is a healing and positive part of life. Sex positivism became an important way to counteract the hysteria around HIV/AIDS, and to fight a sex-negative type of feminism that viewed sexuality as the core of women's oppression.

Sexually, women have come into their own. They are talking openly about eroticism. By taking charge of their sexuality in a way that is empowering and powerful, they have changed forever how female sexuality is viewed. This newly embraced sexuality is not based on a male model, or even on a traditional female one, but on a new vision. Gender roles have been explored, expanded, and even discarded as women look critically at the nature of masculinity and femininity and unravel what was biology and what was social construction.

This new female sexuality is manifest in the many courses available on erotic massage, sadomasochism (SM), how to play with sex toys, how to make your own erotic video, striptease, breath and energy orgasm, and spiritual sex. Female entrepreneurs have found markets for porn produced for women and couples, erotic products, and sex toys made to add to female sexual pleasure.

Female performance artists have publicly explored women's sexuality, putting women's intimate erotic experiences onstage in shows that are often confronting, even shocking. For other artists the new performance arena is female-to-male cross-dressing, with the phrase *drag king* now entering the language for the first time.

For me, trying to find answers to my many questions on sexuality was like searching for the Holy Grail. On that journey I met many of the women who are profiled in *Sex Tips and Tales from Women Who Dare*, women who came to be (sometimes unintentionally) at the forefront of the new sexual revolution. These women reflect the diversity of sexuality that exists in each of us. I respect the honesty and passion they embrace in their lives and the many ways they have used their sexuality to make a difference.

The women in this book have endured periods when they were

denied respect or honor for their sexual journey. In part, the purpose of the book is to redress this rejection and to publicly pay tribute to the contributions they have made in creating a sex-positive world. All of the women in this book have been courageous in their fight for women's sexual rights and have often faced censure, personal attack, and even threats of violence—just as their counterparts in the last century did. Many of the sexual rights women take for granted were fought for by the women profiled in this book, female sexual pioneers who, for the first time all in one place, reveal here their varied journeys as well as their personal sexual tips and exercises. You are hearing it from the experts!

Sex Tips and Tales from Women Who Dare consists of a range of contributions: most are transcriptions from original interviews; some are sneak previews of yet-to-be published manuscripts; others are sexual classics that deserve to be more widely read. The diversity of the material is deliberate, for I believe that everybody's sexual journey is eclectic and individual. The list of contributors certainly reflects this principle. Some of these women's erotic journeys have been so powerful that I have included them for this reason alone.

Many of these women have influenced me directly, such as my friend and mentor, Annie Sprinkle, and Jwala, who twenty years ago introduced me to Tantra. I have always admired the work of Veronica Vera, Linda Montano, Dolores French, and Joan Nestle. For years I have used Kutira's music in my workshops. Carol Queen sold me my first vibrator and dildo at Joani Blank's shop, Good Vibrations, which inspired my own business, the Pleasure Spot.

In my shop and catalogue I have sold Candida Royalle's and Nina Hartley's wonderful videos, as well as Tuppy Owens' *Planet Sex: The Handbook*. I've visited Ky at Sh!, the first women's sex shop in the U.K. Cora Emens runs workshops similar to mine in Amsterdam. I met Minori Kitahara when she visited Australia from Japan. Elizabeth Burton and I have had a longtime connection through her innovative strip classes for women, which she has taught from my business.

The women involved in SM have long fascinated me, and I learned much about sexual power and trust from Cléo Dubois, Kat Sunlove, and Amanda Dwyer. Performance artists Shelly Mars and Diane Tornado have long explored gender issues in their work, while activist norrie mAy-welby has explored *and* lived these issues.

Rosie King has been a constant support, as have my friends and peers Ruth Ostrow and Kimberly O'Sullivan. Much of the knowledge in the public arena about female sexuality was written by those pioneering women at *On Our Backs* magazine: Deborah Sundahl, Nan Kinney, and Susie Bright.

Each of these women is profiled in *Sex Tips and Tales from Women Who Dare*. They also pass along the personal sexual techniques, tips, and exercises that have transformed their lives, my life, and those of thousands of others. These are the contents of the Pandora's box of erotic pleasure. Sit back and enjoy the ride.

Jo-Anne Baker

PART 1

Women Sex-Performance Artists

Sex performances are as old as time. Depictions of women performing for men, or for each other, can be seen in ancient images of belly dancers in the Middle East, in Indian temple performers, and throughout Europe. In the nineteenth century burlesque arrived and the first striptease artists followed. In the 1870s the Folies-Bergères thrilled and scandalized Paris, and in the 1920s the Ziegfeld Follies hit New York and inspired the "flappers" craze. When the sensational Josephine Baker hit Europe, the audiences began changing from all male to couples, who saw this new entertainment as not just risqué but artistic. Erotic dancing and performance went from sleazy to bohemian, and artists gained some degree of legitimacy along with their notoriety. This reflected a freeing up of women's sexuality in a society that was less rigid and more liberal. The same loosening up was seen on the streets where, for the first time, women's hemlines rose and they wore pants, cut their hair, and smoked in public.

Two world wars saw these liberal attitudes evaporate, to be followed by the postwar conservatism of the 1950s. However, in a small step toward the development of sex-performance art, the first peep show opened in 1950. By the 1960s, society was rapidly changing as the first baby boomers hit adolescence. In the West, high employment and favorable economic conditions meant an environment where freethinking and expression of ideas were possible.

After a relaxation in the censorship laws during the 1960s, rock musicals such as *Hair* and *Oh Calcutta!* containing a high degree of nudity were performed at legitimate theatre venues. In Hollywood credible actresses were allowed to do sexual performances on film—Brigitte Bardot stripped for the camera in *And God Created Woman* in 1956, Nadia Garys stripped in *La Dolce Vita* in 1959, and Jane Fonda did a fantasy striptease in *Barbarella* in 1968.

I chose to interview Annie Sprinkle for her ability to expand sexual boundaries by using her real-life stories in her performances of *Post-Porn Modernist, Sluts and Goddess* and *Herstory of Porn*. The viewer is included and taken on an erotic journey that leads to sexual liberation and spiritual magic. Linda Montano has lived her life on the cutting edge as an artist, using everything to take her further into her growth, and Elizabeth Burton has inspired many housewives and corporate women to find the eroticism that lies in the "tease" of striptease.

Sometimes Less Is More

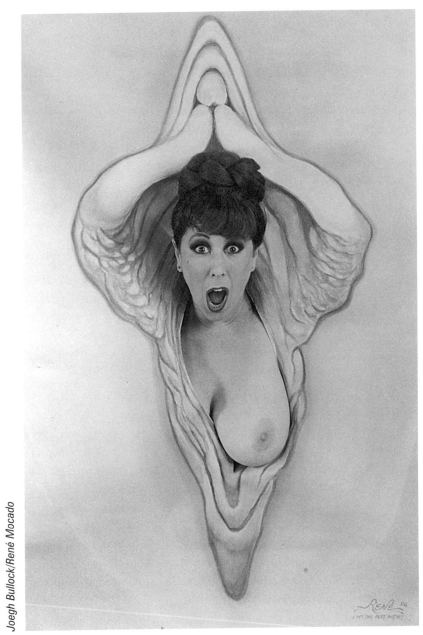

Annie Sprinkle spent twenty years as a porn star, stripper, and prostitute. With the advent of the AIDS crisis, she became interested in healing modalities and spirituality. She evolved into a high priestess of sacred sex magic rituals, a Tantrica, an internationally acclaimed avant-garde artist, a facilitator of sex workshops, a safe-sex innovator, and a feminist pleasure activist. She lives on a houseboat in Sausalito, California.

Annie has taught and lectured at many museums, universities, and holistic healing centers. She is one of the women who inspired the term sex-positive feminist *and is a founder of Pornographers Promoting Safer Sex, organized to educate pornographers to use safer sex in their films so they in turn can educate the public.*

Annie has written and had published over three hundred articles about sex for a variety of magazines, including Penthouse, Forum, *and* On Our Backs. *She has also contributed to a number of books, including* Bi Any Other Name, A Vindication of the Rights of Whores, Angry Women, Ritual Sex, *and* Living with Contradictions.

As a model, Annie has appeared in every major and minor sex magazine. Her photography has been published in American Photographer, Newsweek, Spin, Camera Austria, *and* Penthouse, *and has been shown in galleries internationally. Her one-woman show,* Annie Sprinkle's Herstory of Porn: Reel to Real, *is a play/film diary about her own and society's evolution through the sexual revolution. She is an excellent macrobiotic cook, loves to swim, keep house, whale watch, and take long nature walks. She has traveled the world extensively. Her motto is "Let there be pleasure on earth, and let it begin with me."*

❊ ❊ ❊

I feel I have much more awareness around sexuality now than ever before. I am much more sensitive. I have had a very wide variety of experiences. I used to get out there and try everything and everybody, use lots of costumes, sex toys, try all kinds of fetishes and fantasies. Now I have come back to basics. I am more in tune with the spiritual side of sex, the healing aspects, and the exchange of subtle energies—quiet, simple sex, but at the same time very powerful.

One thing that really turns me on lately is being out in nature. It is so sensuous, especially the ocean. I love going out on my rowboat. It's total bliss and happiness. I love the tides, and the constant change that takes place on the water. Our sexualities are so much like the ocean—always changing, fluid, sometimes calm, sometimes stormy. Sometimes it's high tide, sometimes low. I am not very promiscuous anymore. I like being in very intimate relationships. I like the intimacy that comes with time. I also love to meditate and masturbate at the same time. To medibate! To allow myself to let go into the depths of erotic relaxation.

I have devoted a lot of my life to learning the art of making love. I see it a lot like painting. Each lovemaking session is a work of art! The skills of lovemaking can be learned, just like painting can be learned. I have learned a whole lot about sex from my performance work in theatre, on stage, and in front of the camera. I have also explored different personae by creating different characters, wearing costumes, and exploring different aspects of sex. It's been wonderful. But these days I find it important to know when "not to perform."

I recently attended a sex workshop taught by my friend Kutira in Germany, where we, as participants, could receive anything we wanted. Each person could ask for what they needed, and the whole group would help to give it to them. It could be any sort of fantasy or erotic experience. When it was my turn I asked that everyone do nothing. Everyone stood in a circle around me and did nothing for about fifteen minutes. And it was so delicious and satisfying. I got so high and turned on, and felt so much peace and bliss. Others were amazed at how powerful it was. It showed me that sometimes less is more.

We can be so busy doing a million different things—working, playing, exercising, socializing, and making love—that we forget how wonderful it is to do "nothing" and just "be." One of my greatest discoveries was to find out that I can have an incredible, erotic orgasmic experience without doing anything. Just opening up to the erotic energy available from the universe, saying "yes" to the ecstasy coming into the body. It's just a few breaths away.

In the one-woman show I did for several years, I performed a masturbation ritual. The idea was to evoke the spirit of the Ancient Sacred Prostitute. It was the last twenty minutes of the show. After I did it for about a year, I came to realize that it was not the excitement of building up to the climax, or even the climax, I liked best. The most precious, delicious thing was during the afterglow when I was doing nothing; just being still was the most erotic, wonderful feeling.

Many couples often have just one night every so often to make love, so they will aim to have a big orgasmic, passionate experience. It is not always necessary to make a big shebang out of it. Sometimes less is much more: often the subtle is the most powerful.

I was often busy doing, doing, doing, performing, giving, receiving, putting costumes on, taking them off, building up passion, and being busy, busy, busy—which was wonderful. But I discovered that doing nothing can be the most delicious, ecstatic, blissful, transformative, and deeply satisfying erotic experience.

First of all, to be a great lover you must be able to look deeply into your lover's eyes and not be afraid of what you see. For the first ten years I was exploring sexuality I had tons of sex, but I did not really look deeply into people's eyes. Once I learned to look deeply into eyes, the sex got so much more intense. And far more intimate.

Exercise: The Ecstasy of Doing Nothing (for Couples)

Time: Ninety minutes

Props: Clock or timer with an alarm

Setting: In nature or in a room with candles, incense, aromatherapy (optional), but with no music, or very subtle, soft music

* The main thing is not to do anything, but with the intention of connecting deeply with yourself and your lover. It is not a good idea to do this exercise if you are very tired, because if you fall sound asleep you will miss the effects. This exercise can be done naked or fully clothed. Use an alarm clock or timer to ring at thirty-minute intervals.

* Both partners should lie on their sides, in spoon position, with one person holding the other person. Close your eyes and relax your breathing. Allow yourself time to go inside your own body and into your own feelings. Make your focus relaxation—do not think about particular issues or

plan future activities. Try not to think too much, but to stay very present with your lover. Let go of thoughts. You can coordinate your breathing by breathing together or by breathing alternatively, but don't be too rigid about it.

* After the alarm or timer has rung, reset it for another thirty minutes. Take three deep, big breaths and slowly turn over, reversing the position, with the person previously being held now holding his or her partner. When the alarm goes off again reset it for thirty minutes, but this time turn to your partner, lie in a relaxed position and hold one another. Look into each other's eyes. If you're not used to prolonged eye-gazing this can be a challenge. You may feel uncomfortable at first. Or you may feel fear that you don't like this person, or you may notice wrinkles or that he or she looks strange. Do not analyze these feelings, just let them pass through your mind. Look at your partner and allow yourself to experience whatever is there or not there, without holding onto anything. Hang in there. It's well worth learning to do it.

* You may experience a trancelike feeling. You most likely will go into an altered state, and feel like you are vibrating, or floating, or very light. You may sense a metallic feeling on your tongue. You may even hallucinate a little. You may feel like you've become one with your lover and don't know where your body starts and your lover's begins. Just go with the feelings. It's all very safe. In fact, it's good for you, better than a trip to a tropical island. The experience of being held can be so beautiful. It is a very primal experience and a wonderful way to express love.

* When the final thirty minutes are finished give each other a passionate kiss and take a few deep breaths. If it seems hard to talk, then don't. Or if you're anxious to talk, then do. You may want to share some thoughts or feelings with each other. This exercise can create some wonderful pillow talk.

Although this sounds simple, perhaps even boring, don't knock it till you try it! You might find this is some of the best lovemaking

you've ever had. It can be deeply fulfilling. Your various energy bodies are merging. Your angels might be hovering above you, enraptur-
ing each other. You could have astral sex. What couples can learn
most from this exercise is the art of being together without having
to sexually perform, and you will be practicing how to totally relax
during lovemaking. If you do not have ninety minutes, do this exercise in whatever time you have; just reduce the time proportionately,
say into twenty-minute or ten-minute intervals.

Exercise: The Ecstasy of Doing Nothing (for Singles)

Time: Thirty minutes

Props: Full-length mirror, clock or timer with an alarm

Setting: In a room with candles, incense, aromatherapy
(optional), but with no music or very soft music

* Set the alarm or timer for thirty minutes. Take off your
clothes and, using cushions, prop up the mirror and place
it in front of you so you can lie on your side facing it.
Look at yourself as if you were looking at someone else.
See yourself as your lover. This is a very powerful exercise,
because by allowing yourself to just be with yourself, by
looking into your own eyes, you can create a unique intimacy with yourself. Get to know yourself better. It's fantastic.

This Time Before We Are No Longer Fertile

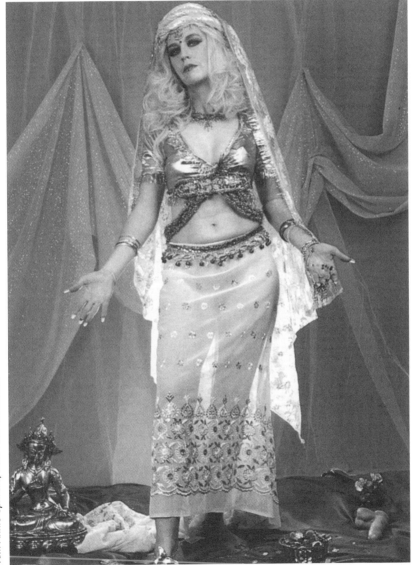

From Annie Sprinkle, Post-Porn Modernist

Linda Montano is a performance artist who addresses issues of endurance, life as art, art as life, humor as healing in art and life, and art as "great therapy." She has been performing her fears, fantasies, taboos, dreams, and life issues since 1969, when she presented a performance-art piece titled Chickens as Art *at the University of Wisconsin, Madison. In that performance, she dressed up as a dead chicken, complete with twelve-foot wingspan and tap shoes.*

Linda was raised a Roman Catholic and even entered the convent for two years. Since 1961 she has been addressing questions of spirituality, feminism, and art, which led to research on Eastern spirituality and experiences in the rich yoga traditions of chakras, Tantra, and spiritual ecstasy.

Linda translated these teachings as suggested by her meditation teacher and mentor, Dr R. S. Mishra (Brahmananda Saraswati). For fourteen years, from 1984 to 1998, she experienced the body's seven chakras, or energy centers, by wearing clothes for a full year exclusively in the color that corresponded to a particular chakra. Each year she changed to a new color, based on the next chakra. When she completed all seven chakras, she began the cycle again. She has also performed Chakraphonics for fourteen years, a sound-based work based on a response to the energies found in the chakras.

While many sexuality performance artists cite Annie Sprinkle as their formative influence, Sprinkle herself acknowledges that it was Linda Montano who convinced her that she was an artist, not just a sex worker. Linda lives her art, so her personal expression is difficult to translate into tips or exercises and instead reflects her internal journey.

✳ ✳ ✳

My most transformative sexual event occurred just before menopause, when a very strong sexual energy flooded my being. It was primal, feral, a last gasp indicating that I had hours to mate before I would no longer be able to bring a baby into the world. It was without reason, and I was led by the first desire. I had no control, no sense of consequences.

Later I read that this is quite common and that this is a very powerful time for women—this time before we are no longer fertile. Women at this time are driven to procreate. I was mad with passion, insane. Out of my mind. Willing to die. And I almost did die. I was driven to the edge of madness. So my advice to all women who are not yet premenopausal is this: listen when you get there, and remember that every action has consequences.

Tips for the Premenopausal Woman

* When you are about seven years from menopause, or perimenopausal, in your late thirties or early forties, note the change in your sexual energy.

* If you are totally, wildly, passionately obsessed with someone who is not available to you, be aware of the feeling.

* Check yourself every time you want to think that you are able to do anything you want, with whomever you want, whenever you want, even though such a thought is not an accurate assessment of the situation.

* Write down ideas for how you can use your tornado of erotic energy in ways more beneficial for you and the world.

* Choose one of these ideas, and either think about it or do it.

* Thank yourself for not messing around with someone else's space or life or wife or husband or career or karma.

* Reward yourself.

Stripping: A Creative Fantasy World

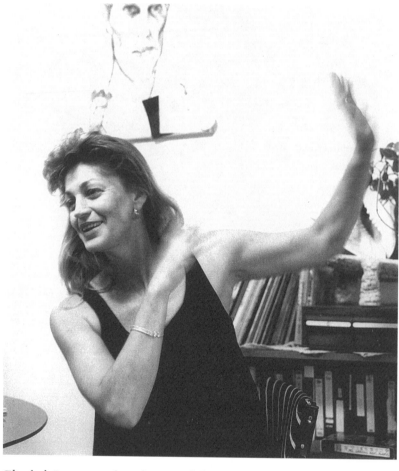

Elizabeth Burton was brought up Catholic in a tiny mining town in New South Wales, Australia. At fourteen she moved to Sydney with her family and became an apprentice hairdresser. One night, a girlfriend who was a go-go dancer persuaded Elizabeth to stand in for her at work, as the friend had a double booking. Elizabeth wore an exotic costume, ad-libbed some dance movements, and when she heard the applause knew that she had found her calling.

She spent the next decade traveling the world: entertaining troops in Vietnam, performing throughout America and Europe in nightclubs and cabarets, and appearing on film.

For many years Elizabeth taught housewives, corporate women, and grandmothers how to get the most out of stripping. She is presently studying fine arts and upon graduation will become an art teacher. She has a teenage daughter.

✳ ✳ ✳

When I first started stripping, I saw other girls being quite vulgar and decided then that if I was going to be a stripper I would present myself in the most beautiful way possible. Converting to Buddhism in 1971 helped me to achieve this in my work. According to the teaching of Buddha, the body is the temple and our instrument, and when one speaks with it, it becomes one's own offering and prayer.

Stripping is a dying art, which is very sad. In the days of burlesque, women appeared as part of a creative fantasy world, wearing costumes and doing elaborate routines. This has all changed; strippers today are struggling to find work. Tabletop or lap dancers have taken over, and there are no classy strip venues; high-class entrepreneurs no longer pay the artists. My way of striptease was to have lots of emphasis on the tease and to wear many layers for the strip.

For a number of years I have been teaching stripping to women of all ages and backgrounds for their personal development, and this has made me confident in my belief that we are all goddesses. Our body is our home, transportation, temple, and the place of our sexuality. No matter what shape or size you are, you are perfect for you. My philosophy is mastication, masturbation, meditation, and mobility—if we did these four things all our lives would be more peaceful on earth.

You can strip to any kind of music, but my favorites are Joe Cocker's "Leave Your Hat On," Larry Adler's "The Glory of Gershwin," the soundtrack to *The Low Down Dirty Shame*, and anything by Aretha Franklin or Marvin Gaye. To do a successful strip start by creating a sexy ambience with low lighting. You can strip out of anything—from a corporate suit to casual clothes to your best dress. The more layers and props you have, the better; use gloves, layers of underwear, a hat, a feather boa, a fan.

Use a shawl to drape, tie, or hold around your body for any moments of vulnerability. If you are wearing tights or stockings, roll them down your body seductively. You can even use a vibrator or sex toys in your act. Make sure your audience helps you remove your clothes. Have eye contact and a sense of humor by smiling and laughing.

Practice in a mirror the moves you wish to incorporate in your routine by holding and rotating your pelvis and becoming confident with what you wish to create in your dance. The routine is only limited by your imagination. To give your legs a beautiful line always point your toes. Practice walking and dancing in proper-fitting high heels—the higher the better—as this gives a very sexy look.

Exercise: A Guide to Help You with Your Stripping Routine

* Start by standing, one foot in front of the other, and stroking your body, beginning at your ankles and working up your body and finally stretching your hands above your head.

* Posture is important: standing up straight enables you to breathe deeply and enhances your presence. When you stand up straight, squeeze your bottom, lift your rib cage, and relax your shoulders.

* Next, place your hands on your bottom with your knees relaxed, and do a bounce from side to side.

* To do the Titty Dance, grip both of your wrists with your hands. Push and relax at the same time. This will move your pectoral muscles and make your breasts bounce.

* Throw your hands out to the side and shake your shoulders, step to the side, and move your hips from side to side in time to the music. Bend your knees, rotating your hips to the right and left.

* For the Big Old Booty Roll place your hands on your bent knees, stick out your bottom and rotate, screaming with delight as you do so.

* Strutting: take a big breath, stand up straight, lead with your breasts (knowing you are a goddess), and walk for eight counts. Freeze in a seductive pose for eight counts and repeat.

* Place your right foot in front and rotate your hips. Bend your knees and sit on the floor, then lie on your back, supporting yourself with your elbows. Bend one leg and keep the other one straight. Point your toes in the air and move your legs up and down, kicking from the knee.

* To do the Spread, lie flat on your back, legs apart in a V, point your toes in the air, and blow kisses between your opened legs to the audience.

* Bring your legs together, recover to a sitting position with one leg over the other, and stroke from the ankle all the way up the body, along the side, cupping the breasts, then running your hands up your face.

* Self-Love: roll onto your tummy, supported by your elbows, and kick your legs with your knees bent. Push up to a sitting position on your knees, stroking your entire body including your genitals. Finish by bringing yourself to a standing position, one foot at a time.

* Between any of these moves you can remove garments, with the audience assisting you. If you follow your selection of music it will help you time your moves.

As women started using dance and nudity to express themselves, the distinctions between the erotic, the artistic, and the pornographic became more obvious. Dance and nudity have gone on to be used by feminists to celebrate the female body, to protest against the restrictions put upon it by society, and to reclaim their sexuality without being seen as simply lewd.

In 1975, in the United States, Carolee Schneeman performed a piece titled "Interior Scroll." From her vagina, she pulled a scroll with one of her dreams written on it, daring to offer the public her interior life and vision. She challenged the distinction between art, life, the body, and pornography, and she has inspired women performance artists in the decades since. Other artists, such as international model Verushka, have used their bodies as canvases on which artists create a human artwork.

A backlash occurred within the ranks of feminism in the early 1980s. Many women campaigning against sexual violence saw sex-performance artists as part of the adult industry that they believed perpetuated attitudes that caused violence against women. In this way, female sex-performance artists, and certainly women who worked in the sex industry, were regarded as guilty by association. Feminism was split, and the consequences of the so-called sex wars of the 1980s still reverberate today. The women who became the sexual radicals of the 1980s believed that the way they expressed their bodies and their sexuality was fluid. They saw that women could control their own destinies to find pleasure; this attitude replaced the feminism of the 1970s, seen by some as relying on domination and fear and alienating women from their own bodies. This led to women becoming sex performers.

Women sex performers and feminist sex workers joined forces and declared themselves feminists and pro-sex activists, later describing themselves as sex positivists. They also started to organize within the adult industry to gain more control over their work and over the representation of female sexuality. They used their political consciousness to campaign for better wages and working conditions. In this they followed in the tradition of Gypsy Rose Lee, who organized a union for burlesque artists in 1951. (Until the 1980s, peep-show artists were frequently not paid a wage. Their only income came from tips.) Performance artists such as Annie Sprinkle drew on their work in the sex industry to make a new kind of body-orientated performance art. Annie made her solo debut as a performance artist in 1985. She performed throughout the United States and Europe and found people who were fascinated by her insight into the sex industry and by how she used her body.

Increasingly, women in the adult industry crossed over into formerly "artistic" performance work and staked their claim to be considered legitimate artists. In doing so the power dynamic between the artist and the audience changed. From an almost all-male audience for their adult shows, these artists now enjoyed a new following of feminists, bohemians, and the inner-city trendy. Their work was no longer viewed as just explicit, but as "experimental" and "cutting edge." A female audience brought a different perspective to the artists' work, which changed and developed under the female gaze. Artists no longer played with pleasing men, but instead pleased themselves.

PART 2

Spiritual Sexuality

Spiritual sexuality is the buzzphrase of the new millennium and has become synonymous with techniques based on ancient Indian and Chinese teachings. The word *Tantra* is Hindu Sanskrit in origin and means "to extend, expand, and weave." Therefore, Tantric sex is a process of interconnectedness between ourselves and the universe, as well as an internal expansion into pleasure.

The Chinese word *Tao* means "communion with the universe," as well as the harmony between *yin* (the night or female or passive principle) and *yang* (the day or male or active principle) and the energy between the two. Both philosophies expand into lovemaking, with the weaving of energies internally and externally with a partner. A *Tantrica* or *Taoist* is someone who has taken these philosophies as the basis of experiencing her or his life.

In the West, we assume that if we jump into bed with someone, a deep sense of connection will automatically happen. Traditional Tantricas, on the other hand, practice techniques of breath, movement, and visualization for months, even years, before they make love to a partner.

Sex becomes "spiritual" when it moves away from a focus on genital orgasms and can be felt as more of a heart-genital connection. Then it becomes something you can take outside of yourself to connect with another or the universe. Meditation through breathing, movement, or light can be fused with sexual energy, and this can lead to deep erotic experiences. The beauty of experiencing a deeper level of sexuality and spirituality is not limited by your relationship status, sexual preference, or age.

Chakras are the seven energy centers of the body, located from the perineum to the top of the head. The concept is Indian in origin and explains the flow of energy throughout the body. It became popular in the West in the 1960s, when meditation and yoga found a new mainstream audience. Knowledge of the chakras can be used to open up the senses and expand the concept of sexual pleasure. Each chakra is associated with a specific color and with specific physical senses and emotions.

* The first chakra is located at the perineum, the area between the anus and the genitals, and is associated with the color red, the sense of smell, the urge to survive, and the fight-or-flight response.

* The second chakra is located at the genitals and is associated with the color orange, the sense of taste, and sexual energy.

* The third chakra is located just above the navel and is associated with the color yellow, the adrenals, pancreas, and digestive organs, and the emotions of anger, fear, and jealousy.

* The fourth chakra is located at the heart, in the middle of the chest, and is associated with the color green, the sense of touch, the thymus gland, and the emotions of love and compassion.

* The fifth chakra is located at the base of the throat and is associated with the color blue, the thyroid gland, the sense of hearing, and creativity and verbal expression.

* The sixth chakra is located between and slightly above the eyebrows and is known as the "third eye." Its color is indigo and it is the center for intuition and wisdom. It is related to the sense of sight and the pineal gland.

* The seventh chakra is located at the top of the head and is associated with the color violet; it is the point of illumination and spirituality.

* There are also chakras located in the palms of the hands, associated with giving and receiving, and in the souls of the feet, associated with feeling connected to the earth.

There are many forms of orgasms and orgasmic experiences associated with spiritual sexuality, but the one most sought after is the full-body orgasm. In the full-body orgasm, sexual pleasure is experienced as waves of energy pulsing throughout the body that can be felt for seconds, minutes, or even hours. Once you have learned full-body orgasm techniques by yourself, it is easier to share the experience with another.

During a full-body orgasm some people experience a feeling of warmth or tingling throughout the body and a feeling of having their system either cleaned out or highly invigorated. Other people see light or specific colors in their chakras and especially in the heart, throat, third eye, and crown. The emphasis in a full-body orgasm is to move the energy created in the genitals up and throughout the body. Wilhelm Reich's research on the orgasmic response focused on four stages: tension, charge, release, and relaxation.

Spiritual sexuality is about expanding the charge in the body for hours instead of minutes before the release, or orgasm. Men who learn these techniques are taught how to reach orgasm without ejaculating, which in the West are usually synonymous. In Tantric and Taoist practices these are two separate physical experiences, and men can learn to control ejaculation to extend the period of lovemaking, and not to rapidly dissipate their erotic energy. They learn to be in control of the sexual sensations in their body, rather than the reverse. For women, the main focus in spiritual sexuality is the spread of orgasmic energy throughout the body, which can be done with or without a physical orgasm.

In my private practice, much of my work is based on teaching people how to expand their bodily sensations by learning specific Tantric breathing and moving techniques. When you deepen your own body's sensations you realize that you do not have to find the perfect partner in order to change your sensual and erotic experience of life. If a partner comes, it is a blessing, but it is not a prerequisite for pleasure. My clients have told me that when they experience more aliveness in their body, their senses expand proportionately, and they feel more connected to the people around them and to life itself.

In this segment the wisdom of Jwala, Kutira, and Cora, who collectively have spent decades exploring spiritual sexuality, will uplift and inspire you.

Linking with the Source of All Creation

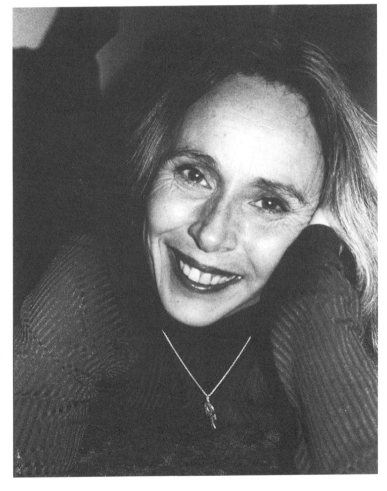

Jan Blankestein/Stitching Amsterdam Photo Art

Cora Emens was born in the Netherlands. She studied to be a health teacher, but instead decided to devote her energies to improving the sex lives and sexual status of other women. She has studied and assisted in self-loving (masturbation) workshops conducted by Joseph Kramer and Dr. Betty Dodson in the United States, and has participated in the seminars and performance art of her best friends Annie Sprinkle and Willem de Ridder in North America and Europe. In 1990 she became the first person to organize and lead self-loving workshops for women in the Netherlands as well as courses in erotic massage for couples.

Cora is a nationally recognized spokesperson for women's sexual rights, with her own weekly radio show, which has broken rating records. After television appearances Cora Emens was besieged with thousands of letters requesting a more detailed or personal instruction in the art of sexual gratification. In response, she made a video featuring a group of women who are learning how to love themselves and how to masturbate.

With her life partner, Shai Shahar, Cora has created the website c.e.emens@chello.nl. They are also the proud parents of two thirteen-year-old daughters. It is to them, and to the sons and daughters of the next millennium, that they dedicate their work.

✳✳✳

The key to making sex a spiritual experience is totally in the eye of the beholder. In this case I would say it lies in the eyes of the person or persons having sex. And that is all that matters. The *way* to attain such an experience does not matter at all. But the experience has such a profound impact once we do attain it, that all we want is to repeat it. So, naturally, being human led us to invent ways to get there. Or maybe we were taught by "higher beings"; only God knows.

We can find reflections of the way or ways to get there in the teachings and practices of ancient temples and in sacred places. Today you can buy books and videos everywhere to learn "how to have spiritual sex." Having a spiritual experience teaches us about death, and sex launches us right into that—"the little death." Through a sexual, spiritual experience we consciously experience how closely related life and death are.

And right there we discover Self—that it is all about the Self, that even the Other is the Self, only projected outward. Some will reach this state while under the influence of sex with stimulants, or through intensive dancing, like old shamans in new bodies. Others may reach it through the disciplined practice of certain (yoga) positions or breathing patterns. Yet others don't seem to need any kind of preparation at all. It comes naturally for them.

I believe it is possible for anybody who wills it to have sex as a spiritual experience at any time, even when the partner is not "spiritual" at all. The big question is: do you *want* sex to be a spiritual experience? And if you do, are you willing to totally experience sex as an earthy, lusty experience? Are you willing to accept your body as your temple of lust? The lust for life is the source of all creation. Are you willing to experience that lust running like fire through your body, heightening your senses, accelerating the speed of your vibration, sweeping away your ego? Are you willing to learn to stay in touch with the Self while all this lovely madness is going on within you? Are you willing to be confronted with your wounds, scars, and flaws? To question your learned belief systems and responses? To find and accept your true Self whether you have a lover or not? You will find a master key there, which will fit any other true heart.

A Masturbation Ritual to Get What You Want

I have always looked at sex as something sacred, something really important that "they" did not have the right to take away from me. It was the key to myself. Through sex I could get in contact with another world that I recognized as "home." I was so happy with this new connection; I could actually touch a button on my body that suddenly took me someplace else! To me, masturbation was a reunion of energies. Suddenly I had access to a world I did not yet fully understand, one of higher vibrations. Masturbating for me has meant learning to play with these higher vibrations. I learned that my body tells me exactly how far to go in containing so much energy, and orgasm releases me from experiencing too much energy to avoid danger to my system.

I am happy I gave myself this training despite the hostility against sex in my parents' house. But I have my load of guilt, which required a long time to get rid of. The remainder I have learned how to play with. I started out really young, but I lost most of my awareness as I grew up. Still, masturbation has remained important to me, and I even made a profession out of it by teaching masturbation courses. I continue learning things about myself, so for me, self-loving sessions can be transformative.

Because I really take time for such sessions—which include dancing or a nice relaxing shower—I can sink into a kind of transformed state of being, and that makes me more receptive to self-contemplation while being sexual. Do not get me wrong; I like to share these experiences with my partner, but sometimes they concern only me. I do not always need him to masturbate with, although that can be fun too.

When used along with the powerful tool of visualization, the energy built up during these self-loving sessions can be strong enough to manifest—to actually draw to you—something that you want. Before I met my partner I had one of these sessions. I masturbated myself up to a very high vibrational state, building a picture in my head of my "perfect" lover and life partner. And he was (is!) a really beautiful man. Handsome too: high cheekbones, royal features, a charming smile, loving eyes—what else could I ask for? But more than that, he's a real man.

In my masturbation ritual I let myself roam in my feelings of lust and in my fantasies of what I would like him to do. I imagined which secret he would know about me instantly. I wanted him to be dominant, to know about my tits, my fire, my capacity, my impatience. Sexually he would play with me, tease me, but I wanted to make peace and give myself over to him in the moment when I'd come, because I would love him. I pictured the man I wanted and wanted to share this with. All my energy was directed outward in one big blast. I came, and all of me cried out in silence, "Yes!"

I met my partner within fourteen days. I recognized him immediately, and we have a very strong connection, spiritually as well as sexually. We live together with our two daughters. We are all happy to have found each other. The spiritual/sexual experience of masturbation changed my whole life. I recommend that you try this at home with practice—lots of practice!

Breathing Opens Up a Sense of Pleasure

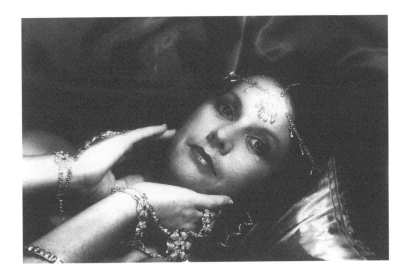

Jwala, whose name means "Volcanic Fire," has taught Tantra in the United States, India, Italy, England, and Australia for the past twenty-one years. She was born in the United States, but has traveled the world and now calls San Francisco home. In her workshops and individual sessions she teaches participants to make lovemaking a sacred experience. Her book, Sacred Sex, *explores positions, breathing techniques, and rituals that are the foundations of her work. She began Tantric studies in 1969 with a couple and became an apprentice in 1970. Her teachers include Osho (Rajneesh), Sunyati Saraswati, Leonard Orr, and Harley Swift Deer.*

Jwala's work has transformed many people's sex lives. Her many other talents include interior and costume design for theater, film, and everyday life. Her company, Goddess for Hire, provides a wide range of unique and unusual services, from redesigning lovemaking areas into erotic environments to Tantragrams, which provide entertainment using sensual dancers, love teams, rituals, and party events. She has produced her own video, Ecstatica, *and appears in the video* The Tantric Journey to Female Orgasm.

Even though sensuality and the art of sensuality have been continual threads throughout my whole adult life, I am now looking at my passion in a new way. Now, during menopause, my sexuality and sensuality are directed inwards. It is a very different experience for me; sex is very intense, but it is not as frequent.

What I do as a Tantrica is to initiate people into the arts of Tantra through workshops, classes, celebrations, ceremonies, and individual or couples sessions. As a teacher of ancient sexual secrets, I am a catalyst to inspire the unaware to go for more liveliness and juiciness. By continuing to strive to become a more spiritually and sexually enlightened woman, I may serve as a role model for others. When people are turned on, their joy is infectious.

Ritual and focusing on conscious breathing have opened the door on my personal path. If I could tell lovers only one thing to remember in bed it would be to breathe, and to make sure they did not ever hold their breath, even in excitement. Breathing opens up a sense of pleasure and prolongs orgasm. Imagine that you are looking at, and smelling, a beautiful flower. Use all your senses to expand your sense of pleasure.

There are a number of key things you can include in your lovemaking, with yourself or with another, that will make sex a more spiritual experience. First, choose a time when you and your partner are relaxed and not rushed, and a place where you feel safe. Speak the truth of what you need and what you want every time you make love. If you want something different, learn to be able to say it to your partner without fear.

If you are preparing for the ritual described below, start by communicating. I now have no hesitation to say to a partner, "Let's try this position," or to say, "Breathe," if I notice he or she is not breathing. I want to debunk the myth that speaking during lovemaking is not romantic. I have watched the whole direction of lovemaking change by being willing to say, "If you touch my clitoris a little higher, I would feel five times more erotic."

Part of this is learning how to say things in a way that makes your partner feel loved and appreciated. It is important to acknowledge the person verbally by saying, "I love your touch, and what I would like now is _____, as this would give me more pleasure." When your lover does the thing you asked for, acknowledge it: "Oh yes, like that." This is very helpful, and allows you and your partner to communicate during lovemaking. We limit

ourselves when we allow our previous erotic map—that is, our past
sexual experiences—to be the only way we can expand our erotic
pleasure.

Exercise: Tantra Ritual for Erotic Sensuality

I have been using a set ritual for twenty-eight years. It has
become a basis for myself and the people I have taught to
go to a very deep level of emotional and sexual intimacy.

* Adorn the room or the sexual space with beautiful flowers,
  massage oil, and candles. In creating an erotic environment, draw on the four elements—fire, earth, air, and
  water—to make your lovemaking a total bodily experience.

* Fire can be expressed by lighting candles, or if you have a
  fireplace in your room, focus on the flames, and take this
  feeling within yourself and into your lovemaking.

* The earth element can be expressed by fruits, which can be
  cut up and used as taste treats on your partner's body.

* Air is felt through our conscious breathing patterns, and
  the more we breathe the more energy we feel and integrate
  into our body.

* The water element is internalized by drinking glasses of
  liquid, be they water or juice.

* Alternatively, glasses of fluids can be used to represent the
  elements: the water element would be represented by a
  glass of spring water; the fire element would be represented by alcohol or spirits, for example a glass of wine;
  the earth element would be represented by a glass of exotic
  fruit juice, such as a pineapple or coconut drink. The air
  element would be represented by controlling the tempera-
  ture with a fan or heater.

We often see orgasm as the peak erotic experience, after which we cannot go on any further. Tantra is about learning to tolerate higher degrees of sexual energy; breathing will allow the spread of this energy around the body. You can even take this orgasmic energy into meditation. By going to different experimental heights you can move from being passionate to meditative and then back again. When you take the energy to that level it is very different from the first biological sexual release. I acknowledge it in the body and also outside in the physical space.

It is important to open up the sense organs and then the chakras, or energy centers, so that by the time I get into lovemaking my sensuality is turned on and the cultivated passion can travel throughout the body. I start by opening up the senses. Because the senses are connected to the chakras, opening them up allows more pleasure to be felt.

Bathing Ritual

Create a sensual space in the bathroom with candles, scents, aromatherapy, or incense. Place grapes in the bathtub and have a glass of fruit juice available. Lie in the bath by yourself for about seven minutes, then invite your partner in and play together for seven minutes. Then get out of the bath and allow your partner seven minutes to relax alone. Do not stay in the bath longer; doing so will drain your energy, which is needed for lovemaking.

If you don't have a bathtub use a large bowl of hot water and a washcloth to wash one another. To be washed is a very beautiful, nurturing experience. Hand-washing rituals can also be performed using flowers or rosewater in a bowl.

Clearing the Mental Plane

Release anything that is blocking you. This can include issues such as safe-sex practices and how far the two of you can go and feel safe with one another. Each partner says, "Have you withheld any communication from me?" Praise and spend time appreciating one another. Acknowledge your partner: "You look lovely tonight. I really like how you have put special attention into adorning yourself."

Sit opposite one another. Place your right hand on your partner's chest or heart chakra, and place your left hand on top of your partner's hand that is on your own chest or heart chakra. Take a few deep breaths through your mouth and allow your eyes to connect with your partner's. This opens up the "love center." Doing so is very healing and centering and allows you to express any emotion, be it sadness or joy. It is also a way of connecting your lower three chakras with your upper three chakras.

Exercise: Kundalini Meditation

The day before I meet my lover I always do a Kundalini meditation to release any bodily tension and prepare myself. This meditation makes a big difference to love-making because it opens up the body.

Time: One hour (fifteen minutes per part)

Music: For parts 1 and 2, something with a definite beat, such as dance, African, or world music. For parts 3 and 4, no music

Part 1 (fifteen minutes): With your eyes closed stand in one spot with your knees bent. Start to shake your whole body, letting go of any tension or frustration.

Part 2 (fifteen minutes): With your eyes open or closed, dance freely, allowing your body to move to the rhythm.

Part 3 (fifteen minutes): This part brings meditation into play. Sit and remain silent, watching the mind, becoming a witness as if your thoughts were on a movie screen.

Part 4 (fifteen minutes): Lie down and feel the support of the ground beneath you, helping you relax.

The Orgasm Is with the Universe

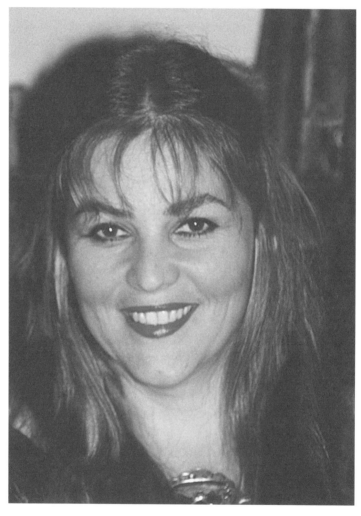

Kutira Decosterd was born and raised in Switzerland. She lived in India for two years, studying with Tantric masters from the East and West. She also has a strong background in meditation, breath work, neurolinguistic programming, Hokomi (body-centered psychotherapy), bioenergetics, Gestalt, movement therapy, communications, sexual therapy, and massage.

Kutira, whose name means "Temple of Love," is an internationally acknowledged Tantra teacher, the creator of Oceanic Tantra, and founder of the Kahua Hawaiian Institute. She gracefully combines ancient Tantric and Taoist practices of energy-raising, music, yoga, psychology, marine ecology, and meditation with a planetary vision and dolphin consciousness. During the winter months in Hawaii, Kutira conducts Whale Adventures in Consciousness with Dr. John C. Lilly, one of the twentieth century's foremost scientific pioneers of the inner and outer limits of human experience.

Kutira and her partner Raphael have been in a loving Tantric marriage for many years. Much of their Tantra philosophy has been practiced and perfected in this period, which they share in their seminars.

Together, Kutira and Raphael have released eleven music albums, including Music to Disappear In I *and* II, Tantric Wave, *and* Intimacy, *and a video,* Surrender to Love. *They live together in Maui, Hawaii, and are directors of the Kahua Hawaiian Institute. Their work has been featured on a number of American and European television networks, as well as in many international magazines. Twice a year they teach a retreat on Maui and present seminars or rituals and concerts in the United States and Europe. They also make themselves available for private couples' retreats, Tantric weddings, and other healing sessions.*

❉ ❉ ❉

Growing up in a Judeo-Christian tradition doesn't leave you much space to embrace sexuality with spirituality. After I finished my studies in Switzerland, I was fortunate to travel to other countries such as India and Nepal. It was in India that I first saw, in a temple, that sexuality can be honored within the spiritual path. It took me a while to reframe my belief systems about sexuality. In the temple, on the altar, I saw a *lingam* (which represents the male sexual organ) joined in a *yoni* (which represents the female sexual organ) as a sacred aspect of the union of man and woman.

The fact that the union of the two was worshipped and celebrated opened up for me other doors of understanding sexuality within a spiritual context. Regardless of how spiritual your focus in this lifetime becomes, until you acknowledge that you are a sexual being, until you awaken and align all of your chakras, you cannot experience a state of completeness, wholeness, and balance.

In the 1970s, while traveling in India, I came across the Master Bhagwan Shree Rajneesh (now called Osho), who spoke of the state of orgasm being the closest thing most humans know to the state of bliss and of dissolving into a state of no-mind, peace, love, and happiness. I became a follower of Osho, which allowed me to explore sexuality in its fullest potential. The master gave me a name that moved me toward learning to accept the body as an instrument of god/goddess. The name Ma Prem Kutira (which means "Temple of Love") was not what I expected or wanted. I was expecting a more "spiritual" name. I asked myself, am I simply a "temple," a constructed booth? I was expecting and wanted a name that was more enlightened. Temple of Love? I had to learn to understand that the body is the instrument of pleasure and of spiritual grounding, which is basically love, but love for the universe. If you fine-tune your temple, accept and love your temple, greater pleasures and higher states of being are possible. Now, after all these years, my body is viewed as a divine temple that holds the sacredness.

Some of the names that we give our bodies show how deeply we are in denial of the sacred parts. For example, in German, pubic hair is called *schambaare*, hair of shame. What does that tell you? Touching the hair of shame. What shame? Where do we go with messages like that? Our language has given some rather bad names to the most sacred places of our bodies, of our temples. In the English language, they use words like dick, willy, pussy, cunt. It's a turnoff, as if it's something degrading. We can call these parts by more beautiful names, like *lingam*, lightning wand, or *yoni*, crystal cave.

These places need to be honored and touched as much as other parts of your body, but if you approach them with a degrading attitude it comes from greed, horniness, or lust. If you touch them as the creative mothering or fathering aspect of the body, if you honor them as sacred pathways of pleasure and love and spiritual union, then you touch them with reverence. These are key things that are necessary to include in your sexual experiences with yourself or your partner to make sex a spiritual experience.

Tantra is an ancient mystical path that offers an all-embracing vision of cosmic harmony. Tantra involves the expansion of liberation of consciousness, making it the fabric of life. The key thing is the heart, the feelings, penetrating into your soul. With yourself, that means loving yourself, loving your body, and accepting yourself fully. How can you love another without loving yourself? With a partner, it means opening yourself up to your partner from your heart and nowhere else, not from your *yoni*, not from his *lingam*.

Your focus is to get into the heart and come from love, and no technique is as powerful as that simple and primary beginning place. Surrender is the key to ecstasy. To allow intimacy and to know that when you look into your partner's eyes, you're looking into your partner's soul. That makes the spiritual experience.

When you ask yourself when you had the best sex, wasn't it when it penetrated your heart, when your minds merged into one, when there were tears in your eyes? In Tantra, the orgasm is with the universe. All that leads to the orgasm is physical, but the orgasm itself is a spiritual experience. There is no sense of yesterday, no tomorrow, only the here and now, this very moment.

In French, they call it *la petit mort*, the little death. An orgasm is like a little death, a surrender into the *mahamudra*, the great orgasm with the universe. When you and your partner are attuned and you connect on every level—body, mind, heart, and soul—you truly travel into dimensions of greater consciousness.

Exercise: Oceanic Tantra Ritual

You can do this exercise alone or with your partner. Dolphins and whales are a source of inspiration and an important bridge to Tantra. Their conscious breathing and undulatory movements are similar to the breathing and movement techniques taught in traditional Tantric practices. These practices move the cerebro-spinal fluid and the Kundalini force (the body's biological life-energy system) from the base of the spine to the brain, creating an energy-frequency connection to God or Goddess, the Divine, the Force, the Oneness. When you are touched with the pulse of these energy waves, everything becomes orgasmic. You can make love to everything, let go of all barriers to pure bliss.

When, after a busy day, I want to reconnect with my husband, the fastest path to our hearts is sitting or lying together holding each other and breathing long deep breaths in matching rhythm, letting go, surrendering into the beingness within us. Our other favorite ritual that encompasses the breathing together is music. Both Raphael and I have been vitally involved in music to create the mood for intimacy and transformation. We actually met ten years ago when I was recording *Into the Dreamtime*, ritualistic music to enhance conscious breathing and the Tantric practice of the "wave."

First, use some New Age music with a definite beat. Start this exercise using conscious breathing, with more emphasis on the inhalation rather than the exhalation. Either lie down or stand up, then move your pelvis, allowing an undulation to move throughout your body. Imagine you are a whale swimming through the limitless blue ocean. Let the pelvis move backward as you inhale; bring the pelvis forward as you exhale. Let the movement become stronger and feel the undulatory movement through your spine, including the neck.

Visualize the flow of energy rising from your first chakra, along the spine, up to your crown chakra, and then back down to your first chakra, creating a circle of energy. The conscious breathing and the movement of the wave create an energy frequency that opens up to the universal mind, the oneness of life. This particular practice, the Tantric Wave Ritual, helps to loosen the pelvis and brings more energy into your body.

PART 3

Gender-Bending

Many people wonder what it would be like to cross gender lines, to walk in the shoes of the opposite sex and experience life from the "other side." Men have traditionally used the excuse of a costume party or a sports-club social night to throw on a frock, push two balloons down the front, and slip on some high heels.

Women are just as fascinated with masculinity and maleness, but rarely have the same opportunity to playfully cross-dress. Many women wonder what they could get away with if they could pass as a man and enjoy male power and influence in the public domain, even if just for a day.

In the collection *Dick for a Day*, women writers were asked what they would do if they had a penis for a day. Their answers were fascinating and frequently hilarious because they touched on women's intrigue with penis "power." Many women used their personal phallic experiences to try to get inside the male psyche, an area that is otherwise culturally off-limits. Almost all of them reported a feeling of power because of their new appendage.

Interestingly, this is reflected in many films, from men's experience of throwing on a frock in *Tootsie* and *Mrs. Doubtfire* to women's taking on a male persona in *Sylvia Scarlett, Yentl,* and *Boys Don't Cry.* However, men's and women's experiences of publicly adopting the other gender are very different from one another. As film critic and historian Vito Russo has noted, when men dress as women they become disempowered in the social world, but when women dress as men they become empowered.

Historically, when women have cross-dressed it has been for survival. Whether they were fleeing an abusive family, a violent husband, or a threatened arrest, cross-dressing and passing as a man have allowed many a woman the social freedom of movement that made escape possible. Other women have dressed as men to have adventurous jobs, such as doctor or pilot, that would probably have been denied them because of their gender. Still others wanted to experience the excitement of running away to sea or off to war and dressed as men to make doing so possible. Marjorie Garber, in her book *Vested Interests*, lists many examples of women who went about for most of their lives disguised as men—from Anne Bonny and Mary Read, two eighteenth-century pirates who dressed as men, to Dr. Eugene Perkins, a Californian physician who was found on "his" death in 1936 to be a woman, to Billy Tipton, a jazz musician whose wife didn't even know that her husband was a woman. Even today, cultural or religious restrictions on women's freedom force some to cross-dress to have the same rights that men naturally enjoy.

Although most people are happy with their biological gender, many others feel androgynous, that is, like both a man and a woman. Although gender-bending is more acceptable than previously—with the androgynous look popularized by designers such as Calvin Klein and Jean-Paul Gaultier prominent in glossy magazines and on the catwalk—outside the artistic world discrimination and even violence continue. This is even more shocking when what constitutes the traditionally masculine or feminine is now totally up for grabs. Sex roles and relationships have undergone enormous changes with the freeing up of restrictions based on appearances and perceived gender alone. One of the most interesting gender phenomena of the last decade has been women's claim to inclusion in the most traditional area of cross-gender exploration: drag. Drag has traditionally been defined as male-to-female cross-dressing, and is usually the sole preserve of gay culture, whose members have embraced their male-female duality. In the gay communities different types of visual gender expression, such as masculine women and feminine men, are generally viewed more compassionately than in mainstream society. Given this fact, it is not surprising that the gay and lesbian environment has most nurtured female drag.

As women have started to "perform" male gender, they have created their own drag-king personae, many with an individual idiosyncratic style. Some drag-king characters have become so well-known that they have loyal female and male followings that travel long distances to see them perform.

Many of these early drag-king performers were approached by other women who wanted help in creating their own male characters. Some of the women were interested in public performance, but others simply wanted to explore the idea of getting in touch with their "inner male." This did not mean just getting in touch with male characteristics, such as aggression and a forceful sexuality, but also giving physical embodiment to this masculine part of their psyche. In short, if you brought out your inner male, what would he look like? For women attending drag-king workshops the answers have often been surprising. Some women have discovered a sensitive New Age man lurking within, while others have given full rein to a traditional male chauvinist. Other women have had inner male characters with sexual expressions ranging from a heterosexual womanizer to a leather-clad gay man. Many women have cross-dressed only to find, often to their surprise, that their inner male is not at all what they expected.

Women get emotionally trapped when they can only see themselves in a stereotypically female way. To watch someone else break the gender barrier and step outside of her or his role is liberating, and to do it yourself is even more empowering. In a drag-king workshop a woman is forced to learn to draw on her own inner resources and throw off her socially defined role as someone's wife, sister, daughter, or mother.

In this part of the book, Veronica Vera, Shelly Mars, Diane Torr, and norrie mAy-welby take on gender stereotypes and blow them wide apart. They explore what it means to act out, even live out, multiple gender identities and how this can expand your world.

Grateful Men in Skirts

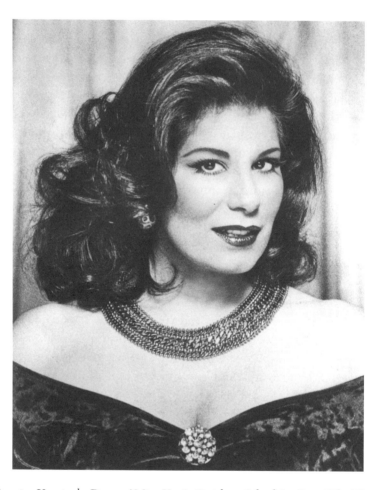

Anthony McAulay

Veronica Vera is the Dean of Miss Vera's Finishing School for Boys Who Want to Be Girls, the world's original cross-dressing academy. She started out as a stock trader on Wall Street, but her religious upbringing inspired her to become a porn star and prolific sex writer. She has modeled for Robert Mapplethorpe and Joel-Peter Wilkin and has also been a cable TV sex-news anchorperson.

    Her political career led her to become a founding member of Club 90, the world's first support group for actresses from the porn industry, and she has

testified before the Meese Commission on obscenity by reading her erotic prose
and showing photos of herself in bondage.

She is an activist for Prostitutes of New York (PONY) in the decriminal-
ization of prostitution. She is also on the board of directors of Feminists for Free
Expression and has written hundreds of articles on human sexuality. Her book,
Miss Vera's Finishing School for Boys Who Want to Be Girls, *is a*
step-by-step guide for male-to-female transformation. It provides a wonderful
insight into her experiences. The following piece is derived from the book's "An
Orientation Message from Veronica Vera, Dean of Students, Miss Vera's Finish-
ing School for Boys Who Want to Be Girls."

✳ ✳ ✳

From the time I established Miss Vera's Finishing School for Boys
Who Want to Be Girls in New York, my pink princess phone began
to ring incessantly. At the other end of the line were the often nerv-
ous, usually husky, sometimes breathy, mostly polite and always
excited voices of the men—the Stephanies and Jennifers, Denises
and JoAnns, the prospective students, all of whom wanted to
explore their feminine side. They felt her like children feel an imaginary friend. Often, she had been with them since childhood. Some
could look in the mirror and see her in their eyes. In learning of the
academy they felt they had found someone who believed in her too.
Most callers asked me if the school was for real. Could I actually
help them to "pass" as female? When I answered "yes," it was as if
someone had confirmed the existence of Santa Claus or, as I prefer
to think of myself, Cinderfella's fairy godmother.

I quickly felt myself riding the crest of a wave of success, uplift-
ed on the broad shoulders of a sea of grateful men in skirts. Not
only had I put my well-manicured finger on the pulse of every cross-
dresser's dream, but I had tapped into the rich mother lode of the
male psyche. Having gone through my own process of woman's liberation, I understood my students as the flip side of the feminist
movement. When women felt the need for balance in their lives, to
share more fully in the male experience—to move from the home to
the workplace, from the bedroom to the boardroom, to be financially independent and sexually autonomous—we created the women's
movement. Men, too, have this need for balance, to share more in
what they view as the most desirable aspects of the female experience: to be pampered and protected, to be glamorous and sexually

desirable, and, yes, even to do housework—many of the "privileges" that we women saw as confining. Cross-dressers are more fortunate than most men because their affinity for the clothing gives them access to these feelings of Venus envy. The Academy offers a mode of action. For every woman who burned her bra, there is a man ready to wear one.

The Academy is my own private laboratory. With the matriculation of more than five hundred on-campus students, I have been able to witness the positive aspects of this unique form of behavior modification. Contrary to what many assume, the student is not "finished" when he puts on a dress and learns to carry himself like a debutante, but rather when he can take the lessons and insights of his femmeself and integrate them into his male persona.

Robert is a student who came to the academy every six weeks. One of our early classes consisted of a field trip during which Robert and I visited a tiny lingerie shop in Chelsea. With the help of the shop's proprietress, we chose some frilly bra-and-panty sets and lacy nighties for Robert to try on in the shop's private dressing room. Our plan was to leave the store with our purchases, to have dinner together, and then return to the Academy where, with the aid of cosmetics and prosthetics, Robert would become Roberta and model her new finery. During dinner I was aghast as I watched Robert eat. He hunched over his plate and shoveled the food into his mouth.

"Roberta will need lessons in table manners," I told him. Robert explained that his professional life as a doctor left him no time for table manners. Eating for him was just something he needed to accomplish in order to go on cutting people up. He proceeded to tell me that his schedule was overbooked, that he did not know how to say "no" to people, and that he feared for his health as he learned of colleagues who had heart attacks at an early age. Here was a man who wanted to dress in soft delicate clothes but was still imprisoned in a tough male hide.

But clothes alone do not make the woman. As I tell every student: understand that when you dress there may be things that you also need to address. I saw very clearly that Roberta, the femmeself, could, through lessons in etiquette and table manners at the Academy, learn to eat more slowly and with more appreciation for the nourishing pleasure of food, and thus lead Robert to a longer and happier life. As the butterfly Roberta emerged from her cocoon, she lessened Robert's chances of dropping like a fly. I am sure that her lessons with the knife and fork improved his skill with a scalpel.

Such success stories are the goal of Miss Vera's Finishing School. Are we encouraging a band of defectors? Undermining the male power structure? I prefer to think that we are responding to a need. The tremendous popularity of the Academy attests to the fact that people want to believe that there is a place where men can learn to be more like women. This is an idea whose time has come.

In those other academic circles, gender is a discipline; in publishing, it's a genre; in cyberspace, an option; in show business, it's a gimmick. The topic has captured the international zeitgeist. Now, more than ever, there is great awareness that gender roles are in a state of flux. All of this reflects the public's fascination and awareness of the current SNAFU (Situation Normal, All Frocked Up). It is the male role, in particular, that is held up to the mirror as Pentagon generals grudgingly acknowledge the contributions of gay men in the military; Robert Bly scores a huge best-seller with *Iron John*, in which men are encouraged to beat the bush and find their origins in Mother Nature; and authors such as Warren Farrell, Ph.D., question the myth of male power.

Remember the headlines that shrieked the scandal of "nannygate" because the women whom President Clinton had nominated for the position of Attorney General had employed illegal housekeepers? More than a hundred years after suffragettes fought for women's rights and planted the seeds of the feminist movement, women were still plagued with babysitter problems. Yet I was housemother to a unique sir-ority, many of whom envied the 1950s housewife and yearned to be in her place. At Miss Vera's Finishing School for Boys Who Want to Be Girls, we do our best to iron out the nation's domestic problems.

Students of the Academy, most of whom identify as heterosexual, are not Broadway babies or drag queens, though that is the level of expertise to which many aspire. The great drag performer, Divine, is one of the Academy's patron saints. Drag queens, who are usually gay, work it every day. They constantly perfect their performance personae. Students of the Academy do not. They are often married and well established in their occupations. But as cross-dressers, they have been touched with a heavy dose of the same magic that inspires the drag queen and made the shamans dance, the power of the combined masculine and feminine energies alive within each of us.

My book is an attempt to bring Miss Vera's Finishing School directly to the reader, with the same care and style we devote to each lucky neophyte who finds his way to our door. In essence, it is our Academy textbook. Perhaps you are a man who identifies as our students do. Like thousands of other men, you may have been dressed in girl's clothes when you were a child, and those early experiences have inspired the creation of your female persona—or, as we call that amalgam of feelings and needs, your femmeself. You want to know more about her. Take a look at her. Help her to be the best she or he can be. The Academy can show you how. Maybe you are the wife or partner of a male cross-dresser who would like to be more informed for the purpose of enhancing your emotional and your sex life. The Academy will help you to do that, too.

I want to help more women—GGs or genetic girls as we call ourselves at the Academy—to understand and appreciate male cross-dressers. I and the other deans find ourselves the objects of schoolgirl crushes from a whole group of very eligible bachelorettes, and we want to share the wealth.

Perhaps you are a man who is simply curious to see how the other half lives. Even a man who has never had the desire to see himself in a skirt can benefit from the lessons of our Academy. In the process he will come to understand not only the ways in which men differ from women but the ways in which we are similar.

A former boyfriend who did not cross-dress once said to me, "I wish I could be a woman for a while. If I were, I'd be able to wrap men around my little finger." I have heard other men make similar claims. Usually they are convinced that given the right equipment, they could be femmes fatales. Here, we welcome all who want the chance to prove it.

Cross-dressing is an act that offers new options. Academy students learn to change their old shoes and take a rest from the rat race. They discover how lipstick and clothes can color their lives. Do not forget that while it is female clothing that is adopted, in many ways the clothing is merely a prop. The Academy dares the student to allow his male ego to be miss-taken and miss-guided.

It has been suggested that men like to cross-dress because it helps them to relieve stress. This far-too-simple explanation supports the myth of the dominant male and grossly underestimates female potency. Think about which values the female or Mother has supported compared to that of the male or Father. Traditionally, Father represents strict adherence to rules of performance; Mother represents unconditional love. On the other hand, men know how to work; women know how to play. And Miss Vera knows how to play very well. Having grown up in the era of *Father Knows Best*, I know that "Girls Just Want to Have Fun." One way to define the Academy is to say that our business is education and recreation. We teach people to have fun.

What you will find here is a step-by-step guide to a male-to-female transformation. Ours is the holistic approach. We emphasize the physical changes, but do not dismiss the underlying feelings; we pay attention to nylons and crinolines, but do not overlook the Freudian slips. Students spend several hours at a time with us, or several days. Courses include makeup application, herstory, girl talk, flirting fundamentals, ballet 1 and tutu, sex education, etiquette, home economics, and field trips (our girls go everywhere!). Most of these are excellent subjects for any man to know, no matter what his fashion statement.

I am very proud of our students. They offer me and the deans—each one an expert in her field—the uplifting support of a tightly laced corset. They are our mainstays. Miss Vera's Finishing School is not all brick and concrete, not even all lipstick and lace, but a living, breathing reality that rests in the hearts and high-heeled souls of its students and teachers.

Students of the Academy, when not dressed in female clothes, lead very traditional lives. Many are family men with very mainstream jobs. They come from all walks of life: professionals and proletarians, young and old, married and single. They come in all body types, and bring to the Academy different-sized endowments.

The femmeself, as a creature of the imagination, is born to be uninhibited, emotionally and sexually. How far the invisible woman goes when she becomes a material girl depends on him. Some of our students entertain the idea that they might live full-time as a female, but for the majority this is a fantasy. By giving our student the opportunity to make his fantasy a reality, we help him to understand the difference.

Our goal at the Academy is to bring out the female persona for the purpose of learning from her. Listen to her voice. What does she have to say? What does she like to do? How does she feel? What does she need, and where will she shop for it? We put the clothes in the closet and let the girl out.

For a long time, I have lived my life as the student, taking in information. Now that I am the teacher, I find that I still learn from my students. One of the things they have taught me is an appreciation of the power and passion of the female. Miss Vera's Finishing School has also helped to balance my energies. Assuming my role of Dean of Students has given me more creative outlets, more assurance, more financial security than I have ever known. Putting men in dresses has enabled me to wear the pants in my own life.

What has it done for the men? Often, even after the orientation interview, a student arrives for his first class and makeover with his face in a tight grimace of nerves. How gratifying it is to see that same student emerge with a grin that spreads from earring to earring. He has taken a brave step. Most of our students have never shared this side of themselves with anyone. It is a privilege for us to be with him at that moment when he is literally facing his greatest desire and his greatest fear in the mirror and to help him see that she is beautiful.

For years, the man who enjoys "feminine pursuits" has been labeled a "sissy." At the Academy, we believe in sissy power. Our students' determination to free themselves and their feelings helps to liberate us all. In his quest to expand the idea of what it is to be masculine by embracing, celebrating and surrendering to the feminine influence, each student helps to expand the idea of who we are as humans. As we step boldly into the new millennium, I am glad to know that many more of us will be doing it in high heels.

Homework Assignment #1: Create a Herstory

Our girls sometimes have difficulty answering the following questions, but some answers they know by heart. They may not know one perfume from another, but our ladies-in-waiting all know what kind of car they drive. Most of the time it's a cherry-red Mustang convertible.

Dear Lady-in-Waiting:

By answering the questions in the homework assignment "Create A Herstory," you are encouraged to see your femmeself not simply as your own Barbie, but as a human with talents, characteristics, and potential.

The following questions will help you discover the personality of your femmeself. Use details that describe not only who you are, but who you would like to be. In other words, your responses can be based on fact or fantasy. Let your femmeself choose the answers. Your responses can be used in planning your classes. Have fun!

* What is your age?

* How do you support yourself?

* How do you spend most of your time? Hobbies? Work?

* What are your favorite colors?

* Which fashion designers are your favorite? (If you cannot think of designers, try looking at *Harper's Bazaar* and *Vogue*.)

* Which is your favorite perfume? (Sample them in department stores.)

* Do you have any gal-pals? What are they like?

* Do you date? Men? Women?

* Are you a virgin?

* If not, what is your sexual experience?

* Is there someone special in your life?

* What kinds of music do you prefer?

* What sorts of entertainment do you like?

* Do you read? What?

* Which is your favorite season and why?

* If you could live anywhere in the world, where would you choose?

* If you could live during any period in history, which would it be?

* Do you participate in sports? Which ones?

* What is your favorite style of home decoration? (Some examples: Early American, 1950s retro, French Provincial, Louis XIV, Japanese modern, etc.)

* Do you live alone?

* Do you own a car? If so, what kind?

* What do you like to eat?

* Do you cook? Are there other skills often associated with females that you want to nourish in your femme-self? (Examples: sewing, housekeeping, childcare, hostessing, dancing, sexiness, making art, feminist activism, gardening....)

* Which female movie stars most appeal to you and why? Who are your favorite famous male hunks?

* Who are your female role models? Which other well-known or known-only-to-you women, living or dead, do you admire, and why?

Exploring Your Inner Male

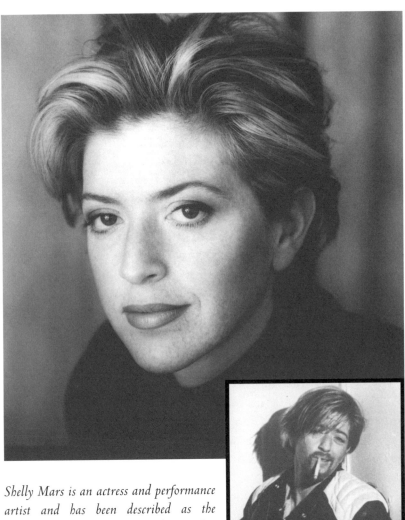

Shelly Mars is an actress and performance artist and has been described as the "Lucille Ball of the 1990s" with a "Robin Williams energy anchored by strong sexuality." She is a powerful comic performer who aims to push herself and her audience *beyond their limits. She is known for her creation of male characters, particularly "Martin," a stereotypical, sexist, heterosexual male. She runs drag-king workshops and teaches women how to access their "inner male."*

Shelly writes and stages her own material, produces and hosts a monthly comedy-club talent showcase, "Life on Mars," and works professionally as an actress and voice-over artist. She has a BFA in theater from Cal Arts, and also studied at the American Conservatory Theater. She currently teaches Performance Art for the Learning Annex in New York and tours throughout the United States with her one-woman shows.

❋❋❋

I grew up as a tomboy, sometimes actually wanting to be a boy and spending a lot of time being around many guys, whom I both liked and hated. I always found some sort of conflict with men; it was almost torture, but I also really related to them.

I think my trouble with men pushed me into becoming a performance artist. My public performance work, as a drag king creating male characters, came out of these feelings. I thought I wanted to be a movie or stage actress, but I realized that it would be more therapeutic to express myself on a more personal level. I obviously had a need to do it and I think people are attracted to the personal message of one-person shows.

Many women feel uncomfortable dealing with their masculine energy. One way you can embrace it is by creating a male persona. I created a male character called Martin as a way to deal with all the anger I had toward men, probably not even knowing the level of my anger. When I took on this character I felt very powerful—I felt what it was like to be in a man's skin and I expressed this. It was sexual and powerful and allowed me to play at being a male chauvinist pig. I realized that this was freedom, and it became very therapeutic for me. I got to play with what I hated and embrace it and own it.

I think that when you do something you fear or have great disgust for, you learn how to embrace it and it becomes ingrained. Most of my characters are different colors on the palette of me; each different character is a different emotional me. Martin is the male chauvinist pig in Shelly. Over the years I learned that all of that was within me.

I think all women can benefit from exploring their inner male. We are born with both male and female sides, and the world would be a better place if women knew their inner male; they would then know how to deal better with men. It is my theory that women can become any kind of man they want. I have many inner males—heterosexual, bisexual, and gay, as well as sensitive men and outright pig males. As I get more sophisticated in working with male characters I have gotten to know the other males that live within me.

To me, it's all about balance. If I'm wearing jeans and a sloppy T-shirt, feeling very boyish for days on end, then I need to wear a dress for a while to balance out the gender play inside of me. It is the same with my work and with my characters. If I play Martin or another male character a lot, it feels hideous—very imbalanced—and I want to do something very different to balance out the energy.

I am not always clear on my sexuality. It shifts all the time, so I explore it in my work. I am bisexual, so I feel a need to sexually enjoy both sexes. When I am around many lesbians I want to be around men. When I am around men I want to be with women. I need balance in my life; I don't like to be around only one type of person.

I love making love with women, and I am just learning to enjoy it with men. It is not something I have loved for years, but now I am learning that through all the gender exploration I have been practicing for years and the work I've done, something has been healed.

Creating these male characters has also been a way to investigate my own sexuality, to know what it is like to be with a woman, to strap a dildo on and have a dick, and to feel like a man in bed. It has also shown me what it feels like to take a dick, to play at being a boyfriend.

Any Woman Can Take On the Role of a Man

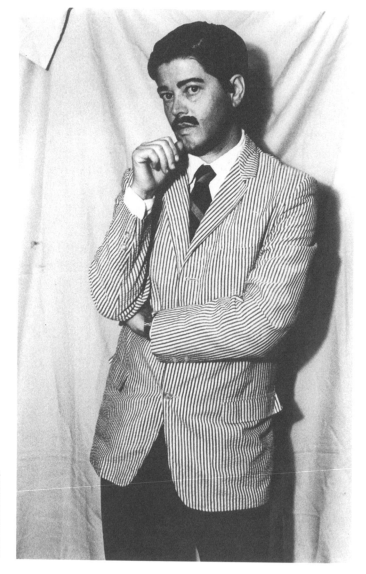

Vivienne Maricevic

Diane Torr whose stage name is Diane Tornado is a performance artist and "drag-king ambassador" who has taught drag-king workshops since 1989 throughout the United States, England, Scotland, Germany, Switzerland, Austria, Holland, and Scandinavia, and most recently in Istanbul, Turkey. In 2000 alone, she gave workshops in Germany, England, Austria, and New York, and she made a performance tour of Japan, where she also taught workshops.

Contact Diane by writing to her at dragkingdt@aol.com, or at PO Box 481, New York, NY 10009.

❋❋❋

When I give a drag-king workshop, it is a whole-day experience. Sometimes it lasts into the early hours of the next morning. At first I held the workshops at Annie Sprinkle's salon on Lexington Avenue and East 26th Street in New York. In a way, the whole drag-king scene began there in 1989 when I started teaching workshops with Johnny Armstrong, who did makeup. Johnny also organized drag-king contests at local venues like the Pyramid Club, and we were invited to appear on talk shows, such as *The Phil Donahue Show* in 1991.

It has been exciting to see how the phrase *drag king* gradually became included in the vernacular and how the concept of female-to-male cross-dressing became part of everyday life. People stopped saying, "I've heard of drag queens, but what's a drag king?" And instead of misunderstanding me and thinking I led "dry-cleaning workshops," people actually heard and comprehended the phrase *drag-king workshops*.

Since the late 1980s, we have presented workshops in many different locales—Annie's salon, art spaces, theater rehearsal studios, private apartments, lofts. I've toured the workshop and presented it at places where I also happened to be performing. I've led hundreds of women through the experience of female-to-male cross-dressing in the United States, Canada, and Europe.

The response has varied from city to city, country to country. For some it has been a continuation of their own exploration, and for others it has been a once-only experience. The workshop has pioneered a way for women to take on a male identity and live as men for a day, or to take the exploration further in their daily lives if they so wish.

I have worked with women of every sexual persuasion—straight,

gay, bisexual, celibate, asexual—and of practically every ethnicity
and age group. I've had a girl of eleven attend the workshop, and a
woman of sixty-nine, and all the ages in between. I would say the
workshop is of universal interest. Most recently I've taken the workshop to Istanbul to work with Muslim women and to Ireland and
Japan to work with women in rural areas there.

For the most part, participants in the drag-king workshop are
women who want to try out another gender. Women have taken the
workshop who wanted to use the disguise to their advantage—while
buying a car, for example, or to gain entry to places and situations that would be difficult to access as women. The idea of creating a male alter ego is a useful strategy, for instance, for women
who want to travel alone in countries where women of any age are
sexual targets.

Some women are performers and actresses and want to expand
their repertoire. Many participants have taken the workshop as a kind
of assertiveness training. Women also have wanted to learn the kind
of behavior men adopt to assume a sense of privilege and entitle-
ment. Others simply have wanted to "own their space." Many have
taken the workshop to enjoy a new kind of sexual frisson. They've
arranged to meet their boyfriend or girlfriend at the conclusion of
the workshop for a night of sexual role-switching and fun.

The thing to realize is that any woman can take on the role of a
man. Gender is not immutable, which means that no matter how
femme you think you are, the opportunity exists to construct the
masculine, if that's what you want to do. And it can be a lot of fun.
In the course of constructing a masculine identity, women learn
other possibilities of being, and this can only enhance your sex life.
Behavior you felt you could never participate in as "Cathy" is immediately accessible as "Bill." Places you'd never consider going—like
a beach at four in the morning on a hot summer night—suddenly
become available to you. This allows for a whole new adventure in
flirting and playing around. Cruising, for instance, takes on a different meaning and flavor when you assume a male identity.

Every woman has imagined herself as a man. How can she not?
In a world where we have constantly been seen as "other," we have
been taught to be a spectacle for the male gaze. What does "he"
want to see? How can I construct myself to be appealing or desirable? Or, in rebelling against that self-consciousness, we've fought

hard to be our own persons. In defining ourselves, we have adopted so-called masculine behavior, such as having a sense of our own space, or feeling the right to speak out and demanding to be heard, or speaking as if we mean what we say, not constantly apologizing or smiling to appease.

Some women mix and match behavior. In a work situation, for instance, a woman might perform certain acceptable gestures, responses, and routines, but in her leisure time she might become someone else. Women have learned, for the purposes of survival, to be observant. We learn what every nuance of male gesture signifies. If you grew up with elder brothers, as I did, perhaps you had to watch out that they didn't gang up against you. For me, this meant developing serious observation skills. All this observation and watching out has meant that women have learned—almost through osmosis—male gestures, mannerisms, behaviors. It is surprising how quickly women assume the masculine; it is almost as if this material is inside already, just waiting to be exposed.

Creating Your Own Drag-King Workshop

The creation of a male identity, like many things, depends very much on your commitment to the investigation. You need a space with plenty of room so you can strut about. You need mirrors so you can be constantly reminded of who you have become. You need manly music, like heavy metal or the Village People's "Macho Man." You need beer, snacks, and, most important, attitude.

When thinking about the male identity you wish to construct, be very attentive to the type of clothing that particular man would wear. If you neglect to think it through, you may feel awkward and uncertain in your male persona. Your outward appearance will convey much about what you think of yourself as a man.

Here is a list of male personae you may want to consider: corporate executive, dandy, mechanic, gay boy, computer nerd, advertising executive, rock musician, macho playboy, waiter, biker, hippie, punk, art boy, academic, laborer, salesman. Each of these male characters has particular orientations that can be explored in sexual play with a partner.

Facial hair is the big signifier in creating a male identity. Even if your tits are showing and you're wearing a dress, if you're also packing a mustache, chances are good that people will think you're a male transsexual. If that's your male identity, go right ahead. However, since other men wear suits, leather, or sportswear, with a mustache or whiskers or goatee or sideburns, you have a better opportunity to blend in. You can get facial hair from a theater make-up store or novelty store. I recommend the kind that is applied in small sections or strand by strand; it appears much more real than a ready-made mustache you slap on all at once.

If you look closely at men's facial hair (and it is possible to stare at men for long periods of time without their noticing), you will see that often it is compiled of different shades. So purchase different shades of facial hair and mix them for a more authentic look. Prepare the facial hair by cutting it into small bits. Use spirit gum to create the shape of the mustache, sideburns, or goatee on your face, and then apply the small bits of hair. It takes practice for your efforts to look real. To create symmetrical sideburns, do them one at a time. Eyebrows can be thickened with mascara, but if you pluck, you may need to add facial hair to fill in the gaps. After you apply facial hair, add five o'clock shadow, but first clean up any traces of spirit gum from the skin to avoid a patchy look. For five o'clock shadow, use a blush brush to apply dark brown or black eye shadow (make sure it has a matte finish rather than a sparkly or frosted one). Don't forget the neck. If you examine men's necks, you'll see that five o'clock shadow is stronger along the edge of the lower jawbone.

With dark eye shadow, you can emphasize existing bags or circles under the eyes. Men don't have the worries women are supposed to have about signs of age and haggardness. A little age may even enhance your male appearance and give you that rugged look! If you have long hair, either comb it back and hold it with a rubber band at the nape of the neck or let the hair hang limply down the back. If you are going to let your hair hang loose, try parting your hair in the middle rather than at the side. If you think your hair still doesn't look right, try adding some hair gel. Experiment with combing your hair in a different style; play around with your look. Whatever length or type of hair you have, you can be sure there is a male with the same.

To bind your breasts, wind a four- to five-inch-wide elastic bandage around the torso, starting at the base of the breasts and covering the nipples first. It's useful to have someone help you distribute the bandage evenly and without creasing, because when you move around any creases can bunch up and your breasts may pop out! The binding should be secure but not so tight that you have difficulty breathing. If you have large breasts, you may need two elastic bandages; they should overlap slightly so there isn't a gap between them. If, after binding, you feel like your breasts still bulge too much, put on a shirt, and you'll see that you've suddenly acquired pronounced pectoral muscles!

There are many ways to construct a fake penis. Some people use condoms stuffed with cotton wool; others use rolled-up socks or a banana or a dildo. You may wish to titillate your partner by unzipping your fly to reveal your "manhood" and playing with this toy together. Or you may wish to have just the suggestion of a bulge, which can also be arousing to look at and to stroke.

Regarding shoes: don't try to get away with women's sports shoes—they aren't unisex. Men's shoes are wider and roomier than women's. Wear extra socks to adjust to the fit. When you put on men's shoes, you feel as if you are fully standing on the earth and owning the space under your feet. The strong physical contact with the ground has a consequent psychological effect. Experience it.

I've based the following observations about behavior on a stereotypical white, middle-class American male. This is because, unfortunately, stereotypes can represent the norm, or at least what can be identified as "typically male." The character you want to create may not resemble this description, but from it you can extrapolate useful information.

It is important to stop smiling. Right now. As women we smile frequently to make ourselves appear unthreatening and so that people can feel comfortable in our company. Men generally don't smile as much as women—they smile when there is a reason to smile.

Practice opaqueness so that you are impervious to even the most penetrating stare. To understand this, watch any gray-haired man in a suit. A sense of power and purpose is conveyed in his dress, body language, gesture, and facial expression. When you walk into a room as a man in a suit, people take notice of you. You are accorded significance without even opening your mouth or doing anything.

You are expected to be arrogant and forceful, because as a man in a man's world, you are right! Even if you're not, never admit it, and don't apologize. Expect to be treated with respect and privilege, and never show signs of uncertainty or discomfort, because this could be construed as not being in charge, and it is most important that you maintain authority at all times.

When you walk, jut your feet out to the side. The action comes from the shoulders. Hips are frozen and are led by the swing in the shoulders from side to side. As you walk, take up a lot of space and let your weight fall first to one side and then the other. In addition, think of your territory as extending about three feet out from you all around your body. Anyone who steps into your boundary is looking for trouble. As you walk and perform most actions, hold your hands partially clenched. Or hang them in your pockets. The arms hang down too, and are bent at the elbow.

Sit with your legs wide apart and your feet planted firmly on the floor. If your legs protrude into another person's seat space (as on a subway train), that's not your problem. If you are not reading a newspaper, rest your folded hands in front of your cock. To cross your legs, make a figure-4 shape with the ankle resting on the knee of the other bent leg. As you sit down, adjust your pants by pulling up the creases at the knees just before you take your seat. Then sink down deep with your ass touching the back of the chair. Never sit on the edge of the seat—that's what women do. When you get up from the chair, take your time. Don't spring up. Lean forward, straighten up, and take a step.

In developing a male persona, you will need to discover certain abilities that you never developed as a woman. Being able to stare "through" someone is a good example. As a woman, when someone stares at you, you automatically look down and avert your gaze, because you don't want to enter into a confrontation with that person unless you are attracted to him or her, in which case you might return the gaze. As a man, learn to look at people as if your gaze is initiated from deep inside your head, and give off a sense of self-reserve.

When you talk, keep your voice low in tone, yet increase the volume. Most important, don't raise your voice at the end of a sentence as if asking a question. Be direct, and speak in categorical statements, as if you have the definitive answer. If your talk is accompanied by appropriate significant gestures, you will be seen as male.

Gestures are specific and direct and used to emphasize rather than embellish. Gestures might include pointing with the forefinger or slicing the air with both hands at chest level—as if illustrating the phrase "I've had it with this job." One gesture of poignancy and determination is to punch the palm of one hand with the fist of the other. This is a gesture you can use only once during a conversation; if you use it more often, it loses power and authority.

Men very rarely touch their bodies, unless it's to adjust their balls or to hit the sides of their thighs as an expression of finality. Some gestures to consider:

* standing with your feet together, lift up your heels and let them drop down with a click

* jangle loose change in your pocket

* pretend to listen to someone, and then shrug your shoulders in a gesture of disinterest

* fold the arms and recede the head and chest while somebody is grappling to express himself or herself

* unbutton your jacket and put one thumb in the waist of your pants, and use the other hand to point with your finger.

As you can see, performing as a man can be quite enjoyable and may push you to delve into your inner resources. Gender is an act. Whereas femininity is always perceived as drag, no matter who is wearing it (which is why it is so easy to caricature), maleness is the presumed universal. This being the case, you can see how maleness seems less artificial. This is to women's advantage, as it is easier to pass in the male guise when we are out having a good time at places we would perhaps never go as women, such as strip bars or go-go clubs.

Maleness is assumed unless proven otherwise. Consequently, even if you feel you don't pass, the fact that you've entered into this transgressive act and are performing as a male is sufficient. You have the possibility to create the person of your dreams: someone who will act on your wildest sexual fantasies—and who may reveal desires that you never knew you had. In performing the masculine, you give yourself the opportunity to expand, to go beyond the allotted "female" roles that have been apportioned to us.

I started becoming interested in male roles when as a young girl I became aware of the fact that my brothers were treated differently from me. Fortunately, one of my brothers (who later turned out to be gay) and I formed a conspiracy to subvert our parents' expectations of us. He would do the dusting and I would dig in the garden. He would push my dolls in their baby buggy around the block and I would make a building with his Legos™.

Later, when I became involved with the feminist movement in London in 1968, I did further research and reading on ideas of gender difference. By studying dance and theater, I became involved in examining ideas of androgyny through movement. My first performance was in 1982 in New York. My character was a Jean-Paul Belmondo type, and my friend played a pregnant Vietnamese woman who had recurred in his dreams. I also created a boy/woman strip act that I performed at various clubs in New York between 1978 and 1983. Many of the theater performances I've presented in the past fifteen years have involved the development of different male characters. I have six male identities I've been messing about with over the years. I've also constructed spur-of-the-moment characters for club gigs.

My public performances involving gender exploration have affected my personal exploration of gender and sexuality. I am much more open to playing with roles. In sexual play, it can be liberating to put on costumes and become someone else. I am very skilled at doing so, and my girlfriend loves it! We both dress in drag and go out as two gay men, or I'll be a woman and she the guy, or vice versa. It definitely adds to our sex life.

Like a Bridge over the Sex Divide

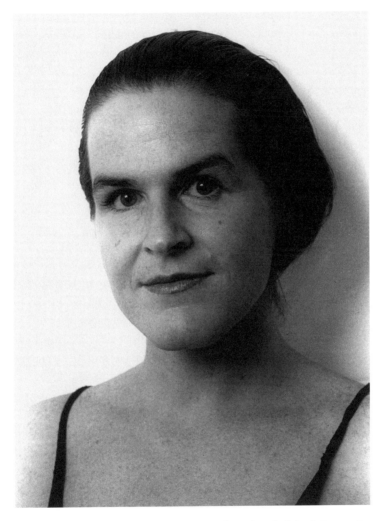

norrie mAy-welby was born with more capitals and a slightly different shape to hir name, which is no less true of hir body. (Since norrie is of no single fixed gender, I have used androgynous pronouns, that is, "hir" for her or his, "zie" for she or he, and "hirs" for hers or his.) Zie came to Perth, Western Australia, with hir family as a ten-pound tourist, in a scheme designed to prop up the monocultural values of white Australia. Since then, zie has since been working almost nonstop to build a culture that values diversity, freedom of expression, and sex positivity (or, in other words, to undermine and destroy the dominant culture zie was imported to promote).

norrie has been a published writer since high school, working hir own bent on sexuality into Perth's university and gay press. Zie moved to Sydney in 1988, joined the management committee of the Australian Transsexual Association (a welfare organization), and became coordinator of the more politically oriented Transgender Liberation Coalition. Zie copresented a radical workshop on gender, transgender, and feminism at the 1991 Queer Collaborations conference, and with hir copresenter, Aidy Griffin, wrote the groundbreaking "Gender Agenda" columns in the Sydney Star Observer.

norrie has written, performed, and taught on gender, sexuality, and transgender in various forums and media, including the Third International Congress on Sex and Gender (Oxford University, 1998), the New South Wales high-school textbook Girl Talk, *and the television documentaries* On Becoming *and* Sexing the Label. *Zie is currently working with the Sex Workers Outreach Project.*

✷✷✷

I thank the Goddess I was labeled a male at birth, or else I may never have been able to find any sympathy for men. It would seem to me, from my body's topography and eruptions, that I even had a normal amount of testosterone when I was a teenager.

However, this failed to dispose me toward violence, rape, or any other uncontrollable passions. Nor did I have any appreciation of the notion that male and female humans were different species, and that exploitation and manipulation of one by the other was acceptable practice.

This idealistic idyll was shaken up when I found my self-expression disapproved and penalized by an adult workplace that imposed gender conformity. My self-expression was classified as "female" and prohibited for one of apparently male physiognomy. To cut a long story (among other things) short, I changed my physiognomy and asserted a female social identity. This did not seem to me to be a change of gender, for I had never had a sense of myself as male, merely a "natural" affirmation of my inherent femaleness. Of course, this affirmation was only made necessary because of a social insistence on either male or female gender identification.

When I was about ten, I had crushes on a couple of girls, but I was thoroughly disenchanted by the gender roles that were expected in opposite-sex relations. I wanted to be treated as an equal, not as a transparent klutz with a fixed agenda to be manipulated and exploited. I also had a crush on a boy at about the same age, and idly wondered if this meant I was homosexual.

I had another long-lasting crush on a boy during my midteens, and consequently identified myself as gay. My initial sexual interactions were less definitive, however, since some of my partners were male, some were female, and my behavior ranged from normal heterosexual male to passive homosexual, to throw around some clinical labels.

I rigidly policed my behavior as a pre-op transsexual to make sure I would qualify for genital-realignment surgery. I sought this partly because I believed the popular notion that one's public gender should be properly reflected in the gender of one's privates. I bought the idea that has oppressed women since the advent of advertising: that we should all aspire to one ideal type of female body. I even came to believe that there were "proper" ways for women to behave, tolerated no departure from this in myself, and took pride in my conformity to ideas of femininity.

I then found I was the sort of woman who was treated very badly by straight men, and I became open to the idea of changing what sort of woman I was. I explored personal-development books and courses, freed myself from the bounds of preexisting self-notions, and allowed myself to express all that was in me as a whole human, without regard to gender limitations. Of course, being a whole woman is not essentially different from simply being a whole person.

When I identified myself as female and lived as transsexual, almost all my partners were male, although their own identifications ranged from straight to bisexual to gay (much as they had when I was a garden-variety gay boy). A few lesbians tried to seduce me, too. As I wasn't bound by a fear of homosexuality (having been happily a gay male), many of these seductions were consummated.

Now that I have grown beyond standard gender limitations, I am not only fluid in my social gender, but I also play with gender in intimate interactions. I am confident enough in my femininity to wear a strap-on without feeling that doing so compromises my womanhood. I have rejected any shame about being transgender, and being visible about this spares me from involvement with sexually insecure, sexist, and homophobic men. I've also experienced the sexual attraction inherent in gender ambiguity and have consummated relations with a few transgender people of various gender types.

I have since found myself at the forefront of gender and transgender politics, negotiating practical solutions for gender-gifted people in gender-restricted situations, while working toward the ideal where no one is persecuted or treated as inferior because of their gender status. As long as there are men and women who think the other sex is an alien race, as long as intersexed (hermaphrodite) children are denied the gender they were born with, as long as people are persecuted for the sake of "gender norms," I will continue to work for the destruction of gender tyranny.

As a transgendered person, some people (and some laws) see me as male, some as female, some as "not male," some as "not female." Sometimes I may experience myself as masculine, sometimes as feminine. Whether I am essentially a male or female person is like asking the planet whether it is essentially a day person or a night person.

Finding standard gender terms ill-fitting, I coined my own term to reflect my own gender position. The term is *spansexual*. The word *sex* comes from the Latin *seco*, to divide, and I span the division. Like a bridge, I am located in both places at once, and I've traveled from one side to the other. Like a bridge over the sex divide, I overlook the space between the sexes, and I can see each side from both sides.

The sexes are not poles apart. They may be on different sides of the equator, but the equator is just an imaginary line. The term *spansexual* applies, then, not just to bridging the divisions of sex, but to bridging any and all harmful divisions.

Society has made many divisions within and between us: divisions of race, sex, age, class, color, and sexuality, and divisions between ourselves and our environment. I believe that we can honor our unique differences without being separate from each other, that we can express any particular aspect of ourselves without disowning other aspects, and that we can live as part of our environment, not apart from it. I believe that health and lasting happiness come from wholeness, not separateness.

I have been a sex worker, and this has put me in many situations that I may never have explored on my own initiative. While some of these activities have not been things that held any appeal for me outside of my profession, some have become part of my personal sexual practice. It was also as a sex worker that I began intuitively practicing techniques—such as channeling sexual energy for healing in a Reiki-like manner—that I later learned were part of New Age Tantric practices. Tantra now plays a part in both my sex work and my personal life.

Having had sex with such a wide range of people has led me to an experience-based understanding of the mind-boggling diversity of human sexuality. Having encouraged so many people to accept and explore their individual inclinations, I would have been hypocritical had I not encouraged myself to do the same. I don't blink if I find myself entertaining a sexual attraction or fantasy that I can't easily understand or see precedents for.

As an amateur, I was often treated as an unpaid sex worker. Once I began getting paid for "Wham bam thank you ma'am," I embraced higher expectations of recreational intimacy. I became much more assertive about getting my own needs met.

Before I began any conscious personal-development work, I saw myself as an isolated being who was dependent on others' approval. I was always endeavoring to meet their expectations and conform to their idea of normality. Since then, I have grown more conscientious about being true to myself, whether or not doing so gains outside validation.

In exploring who I was and who I could be as a woman, I have also explored and developed aspects that I had formerly labeled "masculine" and therefore inappropriate. I have reclaimed and rejoiced in the Artemis within me. It does seem that my current yin-yang flux is mostly yin—that is, female—and has been this way for most, if not all, of this lifetime. I still maintain, however, a commonality with everyone on the sex-gender continuum. There is no fundamental difference between other women and me, or between me and an effeminate queen, or between the queen and a bisexual man, or between a bisexual man and a straight man.

I have chosen to reject sex-negative values, and have been critical of "moral" and "religious" restrictions on physical pleasure and sexuality. It seems to me that these restrictions are designed to keep us from our personal power and pleasure, to make us dependent on external authority. I experience my sensuality and sexuality as divine gifts that can unite me with myself, with other people, and with the physical and spiritual world I am part of.

The more connected I allow myself to be with the seen and unseen energies within and around me, the more these energies flow to, through, around, and within me. The more I trust that the universe I am part of will look after its own, the less my ego stresses out trying to manage the universe. The less division I allow between myself and other people—whether based on gender, race, class, or whatever—the more I experience my connection to all of humanity and to all of the human that I am.

Exercise: Gender Play

As different as male and female bodies seem to be, the similarities are even more astounding. Each sexual feature seems to have a counterpart in the other sex. Yet men quite often have their nipples and G-spot ignored, while women may find their external genitals overlooked. Making love to a man without touching his G-spot is as rude as making love to a woman without touching her clitoris.

Where's his G-spot? you may wonder. Well, I'm talking about the *masculinis uterus* (male womb), located on the prostate gland. This can be stimulated by a finger or dildo in his anus, but penetration is not essential.

The male G-spot is accessible on the perineum, that little seam between the scrotum and anus. Follow the penis down past its base to its root, and you'll find that just below the scrotum, the root of the penis curves back into the body. There's a soft spot between this erectile tissue and the anus. Pressing here will generate the same sort of sensations a woman would get when her G-spot is fingered. (It may be more pleasant to do this with very short fingernails.) You may find it fun to play with gender roles, regardless of the sex or social-gender identity of your partner. Swapping roles can be a way of increasing intimacy, as you actually experience what your partner usually experiences and vice versa. Not every man will be comfortable with being told, "Yes, baby, suck my beautiful dick" when he's got the tip of your clit in his mouth, but turnabout is fair play, I say.

Role-play is not limited to strict role reversal. Lesbians may have fun impersonating a heterosexual couple or playing the roles of gay males, and a heterosexual couple may imagine themselves as a lesbian pair. Imagine that *clitoris* is just another name for *penis, labia* for *scrotum*. And remember, everyone's got a G-spot and nipples!

PART 4

Women Scribes and Educators

In the past, women writers frequently took male noms de plume, to guarantee being published and read. The Brontë sisters, for example, published their first books under the names Currer, Ellis, and Acton Bell. For women to write about sexuality was especially taboo. Yet women have most often been the ones to illuminate a changing sexual landscape and have seen female sexual experience as an erotic signpost of the social freedom of the times. This is seen in the work of such writers as Anaïs Nin, Colette, Sylvia Plath, and Simone de Beauvoir.

Many writers, even novelists, are unintentional educators. By describing where society is, and where it has been, they open up the possibility of pointing to where society may be going. Books, magazines, and newspapers travel, and the ideas expressed in one part of the world can easily be taken up in another, making every sexuality writer a potential educator. Publications are passed among friends, reach a wide audience, and help to spread information.

Previously, primary information on sexuality came from the medical profession. Psychologists, therapists (New Age and traditional), and lifestyle writers are now just as likely to dispense valuable sexual advice as your local doctor.

Women writers also turned their gaze on the erotic imagination, and in the 1970s new collections of racy short stories, full-length sex novels, and feminist pornography appeared. For the first time, erotica was written from a female point of view, with women and men described through the eyes of a woman. Desire, sexual destiny, and fantasies were reshaped.

One of the most important aspects of second-wave feminism was the rise of independent feminist publications and female-owned and -controlled presses. These early women's presses printed some of the first sexual self-help manuals, women's health publications, and collections of woman-oriented erotic stories. Lesbian magazines soon followed, and in 1984 the appearance in the United States of *On Our Backs*, a parody of the popular feminist magazine *off our backs*, changed the public landscape of female desire forever. It was the inspiration for many magazines that followed, from the U.K.'s *Quim* to Australia's *Wicked Women*.

Whole new areas of sexuality opened up for discussion through these publications, and their attitudes flowed over into the new heterosexual women's magazines, such as *Australian Women's Forum* and *New Woman*. Together they proved that a market existed eager for a woman's perspective on sexual exploration and education.

For women who were socially isolated, such publications had the effect of enhancing their view of the world. They were exposed to different images of women, to the work of the newest writers on women's sexuality, and to information about the emerging women's-sexuality businesses. Although women's sex shops were opening, with products designed for a woman's body, it was the support offered by female sexuality writers that contributed to the change of consciousness that made the success of these businesses possible. Before a woman could walk into a women's sex shop and buy a vibrator, dildo, or other sex toy, she had to embrace an expanded view of her sexuality that made her believe doing so would be a positive thing.

Another new development since the 1970s has been the number of female writers who have been workers in the sex industry—from strippers to dominatrices—and who have put their lives and their opinions of the industry on paper. These new female sex writers are claiming ground in the discussions about prostitution and other forms of sex work, because they are coming from the perspective of workers in the industry they report on.

However, just as they have forged new ground, women writers have also felt the sting of censorship and have found their work banned or taken out of print. It is not surprising to see many women sexuality writers and educators also active in anticensorship campaigns. In this part, Carol Queen, Ruth Ostrow, and Kimberly O'Sullivan show how the nature of their work has often forced them to become activists for free speech and educators in the area of erotic freedom.

Being Present in Your Sexuality and Pleasure

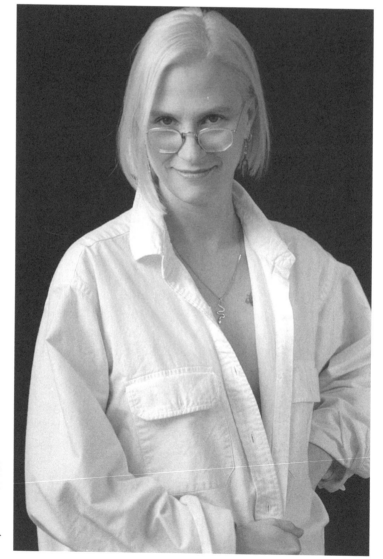

Layne Winklebleck

Carol Queen is a pleasure-activist author and a sex educator who lives with her partner of ten years, Robert Morgan, in San Francisco. She is a cultural sexologist with a doctorate in education (Ed.D., sexology). Her erotic writing and cultural commentary have been widely anthologized.

Carol is especially known for writing about bisexuality, pornography, the sex industry, SM, and other often stigmatized erotic variations. She approaches these topics with the benefit of an academic background, but she also knows them from the inside and openly discusses her personal experiences.

She is the author or coeditor of Exhibitionism for the Shy, Real Live Nude Girl, The Leather Daddy and the Femme, PoMoSexuals, Switch Hitters, *and* Sex Spoken Here. *An acknowledged exhibitionist, Carol has also appeared in several explicit educational videos, including* Carol Queen's Great Vibrations: An Explicit Consumer Tour of Vibrators *and* Bend Over Boyfriend: A Couple's Guide to Male Anal Pleasure *(with her partner Robert). She is currently workshopping a solo performance called* Peep Shop, *based on her experiences in the sex industry.*

Carol is a worker-owner at Good Vibrations, where she directs continuing employee education and works with the marketing department. She also writes regularly for Libido *and* Spectator *magazines and for the* East Bay Express, *and teaches sex-ed workshops.*

Her Web site is www.carolqueen.com.

✳✳✳

I came out as bisexual at a pretty young age: fifteen. At that point I hadn't had sex with any women, but I knew I wanted to. It was the early 1970s, when such experimentation and desire were looked upon as fairly acceptable—except in the gay/lesbian community. I felt close to that community politically, but when I arrived at its metaphoric doorstep I was pretty resoundingly rejected, or, rather, told I was "going through a phase" and that I should "pick one," men or women.

After hearing that enough times, I did. I chose women, partly because I thought I already knew what having sex with men was all about. (From this vantage point, now that I'm over forty, I can't believe I thought I'd experienced it all at the age of eighteen, but I was that uneducated, not even understanding that I had yet to fully grow into my own sexuality.) Besides, I understood intimacy (sexual and emotional) with women as very different from what I experienced with men, even though I hadn't been lovers with any women yet! The lesbian and feminist communities supported me, declaring that relating to women was very different from relating to men. Quite honestly, now that I've been bisexual for twenty-five years and have had both female and male lovers, I no longer think there are such substantial differences. But in any case, at that time, I had to follow where my desire and fascinations led me, and so I declared myself a lesbian and for the next decade had very little to do with men sexually.

At the end of that time I understood that relationships with women were not perfect or easy. I'd also come to understand that I would always have strong feelings for men. They were erotic feelings but also feelings of love—and what allowed me to understand this was the relationships I'd formed with gay men. Though I did not have sex with most of them, there were many men in my life whom I loved deeply. When the AIDS epidemic began to affect them, it pushed me into realizing that by denying my feelings for men in order to fit into the lesbian community, I was doing myself a great disservice. I was not being who I truly was, as surely as gays and lesbians who stayed in the closet.

It wasn't that I didn't love and desire women. But I finally came to terms with my bisexuality in a deep rather than a superficial way. Since then I have always been out as bi (or, as I sometimes say, as pansexual, since I think the term *bisexual* implies that there are only two sexes/genders, and I believe there are many more than that). I have written extensively about bisexual issues, and most of my erotic writing, I believe, can be characterized as bisexual.

I live with a man, but we are not monogamous; we tend to want women in our lives who are in a relationship with both of us. We've had one such relationship that lasted eighteen months; she broke up with us to be in a monogamous relationship with another woman. It's often thought that all bis have, or want, relationships like this—threesomes—and that's one reason bisexuals are sometimes misunderstood. How could a bi person be happy any other way, right? But most bisexuals are probably monogamous (it takes a good deal of skill and maturity for most people to be comfortably nonmonogamous), and I believe that the majority of bisexuals express their sexuality by having sex with women and men (and perhaps others!) over the course of many years—not all in one weekend! Having said this, it is also true that bisexuals have a reason to learn to be nonmonogamous, if they choose, in a principled and mature way. If bisexuality is the capacity to desire women and men, perhaps you could say those of us who have women and men as lovers are experiencing our sexual potential in a deeper way. But there are so many variables in each person's sex and love life that I'm hesitant to make this claim.

Open relationships are not inherent to any sexual orientation; they are one way people of any orientation(s) can choose to structure relationships. And having what is sometimes called a "responsible nonmonogamous" orientation to relationships is not the same as indiscriminate promiscuity; promiscuity is a choice anyone might make, as are celibacy and monogamy. I should point out that promiscuity isn't always "indiscriminate"! Someone may want lots of sex with lots of partners, yet still be choosy about whom she or he will or won't have sex with, and what kind of sex she or he will have.

Anyone who has read my nonfiction or heard me speak about sex knows that I started out very shy—with lots of adventurous fantasies and desires, but very hesitant about finding ways to make them come true. I was nearly tongue-tied in bed, and many of my earliest sexual experiences were much the worse for it. But I was not happy this way. I knew sex would be better and I would be happier if I could get over my intense reticence. My first serious girlfriend helped me enormously; we were together for five years, long enough to get comfortable with talking, sharing, and exploring fantasies, and with getting a little exhibitionistic.

After coming to San Francisco I began to explore group sex, where I met my next two partners, both bisexual men. Coming out as bisexual, exploring SM, working in the sex industry, and doing all the other things I've done, including studying sexology, have situated me sexually in a far different place from the one I started out in—yet I can still recognize that girl whose wild fantasies have finally been lived out. Getting here was a long, step-by-step process, most of it, I'm happy to say, very pleasurable.

Here is the most important thing I've learned on this journey: communicating is enormously important. If you can't do it, trouble will probably follow! But learning to communicate (about sex, about everything) is step-by-step, too, and it helps very much if you and your partner really want to be compatible and happy sexually and—this is quite important—if you don't have too many preconceived ideas about what that means. I refer here especially to rigid, gender-based ideas of what is appropriate for men or women. In real life, our skills and interests may be shaped by gender roles, but often we cross that imaginary line, and it's okay to do so; it's much healthier than being restricted because "women aren't interested in that" or "men don't act that way."

It is also not useful to compare yourself to others. It's hard not to—for one thing, that's what the whole emphasis on being sexually "normal" is all about, which only engenders judgment and bias and even self-hatred. This sort of comparison is, I think, a root of women's and men's physical self-esteem problems. We often don't feel adequate and attractive because we compare ourselves with people in magazines, in advertisements, in movies. A hard lesson to learn is that often our partner wants us just the way we are, but we can get so hung up on not looking the way we think we should that it gets in the way of our sexual feelings and responses. Being present in your sexuality and pleasure is absolutely more attractive and erotically compelling than having a "perfect" body.

These sorts of role-based assumptions and failures to communicate help power the sex industry, in which partnered men pay others to give them what they think (sometimes correctly, other times not) their wives won't. The sex industry is used by single men too, but I know that a good percentage (almost certainly the majority) of my customers have wives or partners. If we can get over the sexual and gender double standards so that people can relate sexually on an equal basis, much of the sex industry would lose its relevance—or change to something not only men but women and partners could and would access.

I honor the sex industry; among other things, it gets (some) people's needs met and facilitates exploration, and the women and men who work in it are often courageous and extraordinary people. But I do not honor the fact that it is set up principally for men's entertainment. I urge women to ask themselves the following: If I had the money, knew where to call a woman or a man to pleasure or entertain me, and knew it was safe to do so, what would I do? If you can't answer that, why not?

A final thing I have learned is if you can't give yourself pleasure, if your sexuality is not centered in yourself, it's hopeless (and rather dangerous) to expect someone else to come along and awaken you like Prince Charming does Sleeping Beauty. Sometimes partners may awaken us, but they do not infuse us with sexuality. It is in each of us all along. Fantasy and self-pleasure can get you in touch with who you are, regardless of who your partner is, who you are with him or her, or whether you have a partner at all. I think we not only have the option of exploring ourselves in this way, but we have a responsibility to do so, because we're then better able to communicate what we want and to take care of ourselves. Besides, it's so lonely and hopeless to think pleasure is only in our lives when someone else brings it to us. Pleasure can be with us every day.

Tips on Exhibitionism

Here's what I'd recommend for someone who wants to get more comfortably exhibitionistic.

* First, show off for yourself. Pick a comfortable room where you have privacy, a mirror, and enough room to move around. Turn the lights low or light candles if you like, but make sure you can still see. Put on sexy music that you like to dance to, and begin to move. Concentrate on how your body feels; even if you wouldn't feel comfortable in public with pelvic thrusts and lots of hip-swaying, do it here.

* Watch yourself in the mirror from time to time. Look for evidence of your own pleasure in the movement. Get into it, and appreciate how you look when you're in your body and happy to be there. Now, begin to take off your clothes. Make it slow, which looks sexier than flinging them off. The slower, the better. Tease and take all the time in the world. Reveal, then cover; now do it again. Keep moving to the music, although there's no need to full-on dance while stripping; that can get rather complicated. Just keep some sway, some movement to it.

* Watch yourself at least some of the time, and not too judgmentally. Be playful. For now, you are the only voyeur.

✳ Now, recline on a bed, big chair, or sofa, still in view of the mirror. Touch yourself erotically. If you want, do it until you come (and by "do it," I mean do anything you'd ordinarily do to pleasure yourself). If you're not in the habit of masturbating/self-loving, I'd suggest you read Dr. Betty Dodson's wonderful book *Sex for One* and then come back to this exercise.

✳ Look at yourself in the mirror—your face as well as your hands and vulva. Watch arousal build. This can be quite erotic—and it is what your chosen voyeur will see if you decide to do this for or with someone else! Take all the time you can spare to do this—thirty minutes is probably a bare minimum if you are going to do the movement and touching exercises all at once. (You can do them separately if you wish.) But longer is better. Among other things, when you add self-pleasuring to this exercise, you are rein-forcing yourself with erotic pleasure. The more time you allow, the more you will trust in your own eroticism.

✳ The next step (which need not happen right away!) is to do this for or with someone else. If it makes you feel braver to have your partner do it along with you, ask him or her to join you. The self-pleasuring part, especially, can be enormously hot for couples to do together. For more suggestions (including what to do if you don't already have an adventuresome partner), see my book *Exhibitionism for the Shy*, which offers practical advice on the fine arts of dressing up, showing off, role-playing, and talking dirty.

Permission to Be Who We Already Are

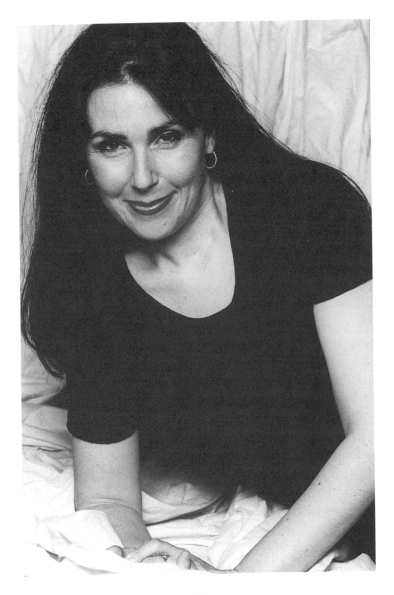

Ruth Ostrow has been a writer and journalist for over fifteen years. During the turbulent 1980s and while working for the Australian Financial Review, *she interviewed Australia's top business leaders for her book* The New Boy Network, *which revealed the psychology and secrets of success of powerful men and became a national best-seller.*

After a stint as the Tel Aviv editor of the Israel Economist, *Ruth moved to New York, where she witnessed profound changes in the male-dominated corporate culture. This experience ultimately led to her writing about the men's movement and about the impact the gender revolution has had on male-female relationships.*

On her return to Australia, Ruth became a social commentator, columnist, and satirist for the newspaper the Australian, *combining her quirky sense of humor with her years of journalistic experience. Then she joined the News Limited papers, where she writes her own national weekly page on sexuality and relationships. She also hosts her own top-rated national radio show. The following extract is adapted from the introduction to her book* Burning Urges: Australia's Sexual Fantasies *(Sydney: Pan Macmillan, 1997).*

I remember clearly the experience of going through therapy. I went in a confused and very anxious young woman and emerged each week feeling a little better about myself. Despite the tears and the pain that therapy inevitably elicited, each month brought me closer to happiness until I started feeling good, then wonderful, and then as if I could do or be anything I so desired. Eventually, I walked out with such a profound feeling of self-confidence, exuberance, and empowerment that the effects have endured a decade later.

Recently I visited my therapist to ask the secret of her success. She explained that her formula was simple. She merely gave me and her other clients permission to be who we already are. She freed us by helping cut away the prescriptions of who we should be and what we should be doing, thinking, and feeling that had been hung on us by parental desire, peer pressure, and social expectation. She allowed us to rejoice in and celebrate the essences of our personalities and bodies, and in so doing, allowed us to become the best we could be.

Hers was a message of self-acceptance and liberation: liberation from the deep resentment and self-loathing, disappointment, envy, guilt, fear, and regret that plague so many of us.

One thing I carried away from her was a burning desire to take her message to others. She had taught me that I could do and be anything I wanted. What I most wanted to be was a liberator—a person who gave others the same permission she had given me, permission denied to so many by judgmental teachers, parents, and various authority figures. Permission to follow your own calling. Permission to be.

This is what motivated me to put together *Burning Urges*, a compilation of people's secret sexual fantasies and inner worlds. In 1996, the News Limited Sunday newspapers across Australia—for whom I work as a journalist—ran "The Great Australian Sex and Relationships Survey" for me so I could glean statistical information on Australian interpersonal behavior. In less than three weeks we received just under ten thousand responses.

I was astounded, not only by the revelations buried in the letters but also because so many respondents thanked me for allowing them to express and unburden themselves. Many stated that they had kept all these thoughts bottled up and had felt tormented or guilty about having them. They explained that releasing and sharing them had liberated and excited them.

I decided to see if I could duplicate the success of my earlier inquiries by putting a small advertisement at the bottom of my column in these same newspapers, asking for people to report their sexual fantasies for a book I planned to compile. Again, I was immediately swamped with letters. In under two weeks I had received the equivalent of two books full of erotica. And what was revealed were the stunning, strange, and bizarre thoughts that lurk in all of our minds. From my largely middle-class readers came a panty-sniffer who fancies old ladies, a happy wife who is obsessed by the idea of exposing her genitals, a happily married man and father who gets sexually aroused imagining a lighted cigarette inserted up his bum. Another gets off fantasizing his wife is kidnapped by thugs and gang-banged.

The following letter came with a photo of nappies (diapers) on a clothesline:

> Dear Ruth, I am an average, 75-kg Australian male. I do not smoke nor drink alcohol. I have a high-pressure job and, as you see from my photos, I have very different sexual fantasies, which I put into real life. I have high sexual pleasure in wearing nappies and plastic pants at home. It is

also a real turn-on to see a partner in her nappy and plastic
pants walking around the house. . . .

Many average Australian men fantasized about watching their
wives go with other men in threesomes, only to reveal later in the
fantasy that the latent wish was to be anally penetrated themselves.
Just as many happily married, rugged, outdoorsy Australian men and
fathers secretly dressed up in women's clothing and imagined they
were women while having sex.

> My fantasy is to wear nylons, nail polish, and high heels
> while having sex. I love the feel of nylon on my feet, which
> are about a size seven and are sexy, and to see my nails with
> pink polish . . . fuck . . . it turns me on just writing this!

Such revelations, I believe, help redefine "normality," and in
doing so, allow us more freedom to be. They confront the way we
perceive masculinity. From these admissions we can see that it is
impossible to embrace the stereotype that "all men desire tall, leggy
blondes with large breasts." In their secret thoughts men desire
other men, men dressed as women, fat women, older women, dirty
women with sexy smells, horny, raunchy women with body hair and
foul mouths. One pensioner, married for decades, craves a large,
black, African male in drag. The world of sexual fantasy knows no
boundaries and pays little homage to stereotypical aesthetics. And it
is certainly free of any hint of political correctness.

Women, too, are a surprising lot. The letters I received were full
of happy mothers and wives who want to be consumed by vampires,
drink blood and urine, have lesbian mistresses strap them up and
torture them to orgasm, take part in lesbian orgies, or watch their
husbands or partners being screwed by other men. I have always
maintained that women are as dirty and pornographic as men. It's
just that we've been unable to express it. Common wisdom has
always maintained that women have romantic fantasies while men's
fantasies are more sexual.

As a woman, I have both. My daydreams are very romantic, clas-
sic Mills and Boon. They may become sexual, but are more often
satiated by a fantasy kiss with some unobtainable *objet d'amour*. I
know instinctively that they are about my need for validation and
acceptance, probably a bit of escapism in the face of domesticity,

and a natural female yearning for high drama that started in my teenage years.

The second type of fantasy I have is the sexual fantasy, which is your garden-variety perverse journey into the undergrowth of the mind. And mine is as graphic and pornographic as any male fantasy I have ever read.

So, in homage to my therapist, I feel I have put together a work that will ultimately liberate. *Burning Urges* contains material that is a profound challenge to all the acceptable faces we present as mothers, fathers, employees, and children. It is not about the side we present that makes society comfortable and complies with the rules, but our most hidden, secret places. Who we are when we dream, when we yearn, when we fear, when we grieve, when we confront death, when we orgasm. It is a book about our pain, our pleasure, our unquenchable appetites and strange lusts. The primal and primitive side of human nature—the rebellious, the perverse, the angry and untamable side.

It is about the hurt child and the wounded animal who live beneath the churchgoing facade. The sexual, sensual, lascivious creature that many conservative thinkers have for so long tried to deny. It is about the parts of ourselves that we must learn to love and accept if we are ever to be free.

It is interesting that many conservative thinkers have always told us that only barbaric or warped individuals enjoy watching pornography or have dirty thoughts. And yet the profile of my correspondents belies that. Those riddled with pornographic fantasies are not lonely, isolated, dirty old men in raincoats or women without love. A large percentage of my respondents are not only married, but happily so. Many have children and share a loving family and religious life together. Many also share their fantasies with their partners as a tool to keep their relationship hot and spicy.

Respected American writer Erica Jong, in her autobiography, *Fear of Fifty*, says her current and third marriage is successful where her other marriages failed for one reason. She has a new habit of writing down her sexual fantasies and reading them to her husband. She claims this is a potent ingredient that helps to preserve sexual arousal and passion in the marriage and to enrich communication.

Having grown up with Nancy Friday and now working on my own body of research, I can safely say that none of us are wrong for having our fantasies, no matter how bizarre or questionable. I have long believed that sexual fantasies are gateways to our fears, our motivations, and our childhoods. They are rich in symbolism—and the symbols can be used as a tool to unlock the psyche.

The sexual fantasy, like the dream, is a compilation of subconscious messages and buried feelings. And these fantasies are about far more than sex. They are about what frightens or eludes us, what we crave or regret, but ultimately—like the sleeping dream—what we need to resolve about our complex lives.

I have always believed that if you understand a person's sexual fantasy, you at once find the key to his or her innermost being. The motivation. The raison d'être. You find clues to childhood. The true state of mind. Here are some examples from the letters I received.

> I recall from my teenage years finding it very difficult to get to sleep unless I thought about extreme violence towards women, mostly thrusting a sword into [a woman's] vagina. I had always been very shy with girls, had an unusually strong-willed mother and an emotionally cold father.

> I have never actually been violent with a partner and cannot think of any reason why I ever would. My strong mother used emotional blackmail as a matter of course to get her own way. I could feel her intense anger very deeply, and experience churning in my solar plexus.

If this doesn't make my point, here is another very telling fantasy from a woman who fantasizes about her man and herself in a ménage à trois with another woman.

> Sometimes I change roles and become the man attending to me or her; then I can change and become her. All parts are interchangeable. This used to trouble me. Was I insecure? Was I jealous? Did my jealousy or envy for the woman translate into pleasure? Was it pain becoming pleasure? Trying to resolve rejection by becoming my rival?

Our fantasies tell us so much, and yet they are a tool undervalued by the helping professions because analyzing them entails the discomforting and thorny issue of sex. In my experience of trying to find a therapist, I found few who wanted to go down this path.

I think it most ironic that sleeping dreams have been elevated to such a lofty status that Jungian dream analysis is almost a science. Yet sexual fantasies—the waking personification—which are steeped in Oedipal yearnings and unresolved issues and needs, often confound or embarrass many in the helping professions. Thankfully, I found a therapist who paid homage to this inner world. She was not shocked or alarmed by some of the things my mind dug up. She found me neither perverse nor bizarre; rather, she used my fantasies to help me unlock my deepest feelings about myself, my parents, my surroundings.

What I discovered was that my head was like a jukebox—full of fantasies waiting to be played. And that I had been using sexual fantasies for years as a way of inadvertently dealing with, or making sense of, my world. If I was feeling a little powerless, I would fantasize about taking control. If I felt overburdened by power, responsibility, and control, I would lapse into a world where power was taken from me, much like judges and politicians who frequent SM haunts. In short, I was using fantasies almost as a balancing tonic to help me come back to an equilibrium.

And if fantasies are indeed a healing tool or a psychological indicator, a grab for power, a need for validation, then I certainly watched mine change throughout therapy as I struggled to come to terms with many feelings. I saw anger at my parents translate into fantasies concerning authority figures; insecurity led to my waking dreams being filled with "conquering" imagery. I experienced fantasies about other women as I struggled to love myself, to hatch out my own identity separate from my mother. I yearned to crawl back into the womb and then to break free from it.

After my time on the therapy couch and now after putting together *Burning Urges*, I have very much come to see sexual fantasies as a journey into self. A release valve. A medicine of sorts, but best of all, a silent teacher. A teacher directing us to our inner wisdom.

While the wowser element of society has tried to intimidate us into suppressing this healing and self-educational process on the basis that fantasies will lead to aberrant behavior, many psychologists and researchers I interviewed now confirm that fantasies are not necessarily things we actually want to do. Often, they are just the opposite. For many, they are simply a cathartic experience that can be mentally rejected the moment after orgasm.

For instance, many women have rape or abuse fantasies for a variety of reasons. But in such a fantasy, the fantasizer remains in control, the one to turn off the images at whim, change events, increase or decrease the tension. A woman can play out a past trauma or her worst fears or most forbidden yearnings, yet she can stop the fantasy, redress the balance, play either role, and identify with either party to quell her anxiety. She has the control button.

One of the most curative effects of fantasies are that they allow us to explore different roles, obsessions, or fixations with impunity and in the safety of our own heads. We are empowered by our own ability to direct and command events, so rare in real life and in the murky waters of interpersonal relationships.

Even better, fantasies lead us to such explosive and marvelous orgasms, with a partner or alone! That is one more fantastic benefit, not to be overlooked. Sexual fantasies are the ultimate safe sex.

Exercise: Exploring Your Fantasies

Find a slot of thirty minutes or longer when you will not be interrupted. Take the phone off the hook. Do whatever ritual will relax you and free your mind of the day's stresses: meditate, run a warm bath, light candles, play some music, crawl into bed with some favorite erotica.

Now, let your mind roam about till a sexual fantasy starts to formulate. Let the fantasy unfold however it seems to want to. Resist any temptation to censor your mind or to stop the visual process, no matter how "kinky" or "weird" or "sick" your inner censor tries to tell you your fantasy is. Masturbate, if you wish, or simply enjoy the motion picture running in your head.

Allow the fantasy to reach its natural conclusion, or stop whenever you feel ready to. Play with the fantasy over the next days and weeks: elaborate on it and add variations, or simply let it go and move on to the next fantasy; consider writing it down or sharing it with your partner, or simply enjoy it as part of a private inner world that only you have privy to. Use this exercise to enhance your sex life to include more of what you want to change and develop. It can also help to stop elements that you feel are detrimental. Fantasy is a safe way to learn to expand your sexual boundaries.

KIMBERLY O'SULLIVAN

A Warrior with Words

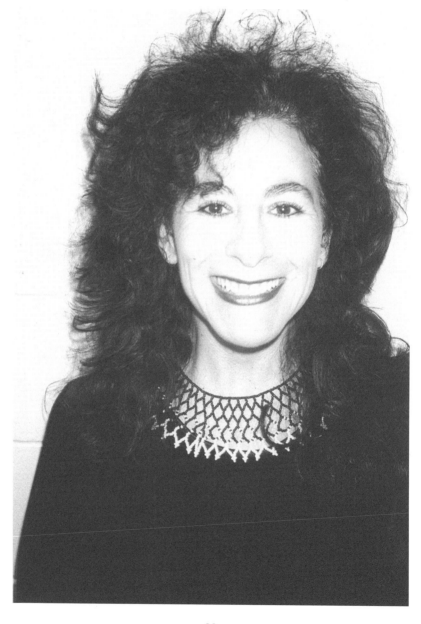

Kimberly O'Sullivan is an activist for social justice. She has worked in the left, the union movement, the women's movement, and for gay and lesbian liberation. She is most well-known for her sexual libertarian views, public speaking, hands-on sex-toy workshops for women, and extensive writing on sexual hypocrisy, sexual freedom, and the sexual empowerment of women. She has been published widely in the alternative, sex, and mainstream presses. Her work has appeared in anthologies, and she has hosted her own radio show and been a university guest lecturer.

For two years Kimberly was the editor of Wicked Women, *Australia's only lesbian sex magazine. She was the first woman elected to the Sydney Mardi Gras Hall of Fame in 1992, and despite being unable to ride a motorbike, she was one of the founders of Dykes on Bikes. A journalist and editor for twenty years, she is also a qualified archivist and historian and has a long-standing interest in the hidden history of cultural minority groups and erotic outlaws. Kimberly's life has taken her in a new direction: she is now celebrating her sexuality and passion for life with her new (male) husband.*

✳✳✳

I have been writing and politically agitating about sex since 1985, and it has affected my life in ways I could never have imagined. It has done great things for me. I have had amazing experiences and met wonderful (and bizarre) people who have given me a depth of knowledge about sexuality that most people only dream of. It has made me a more compassionate person—certainly less judgmental—and increasingly it has made me see sexuality as an incredibly precious gift. I have seen people's lives destroyed because of sexual secrets and oppression, and I have seen people heal deep parts of themselves through sexual connection.

Along the way I have had every sort of sex I ever wanted, fulfilled most of my sexual fantasies, and had some toe-curling nights that will take me to my grave with a smile on my face. I have also endured the frustration of lesbian bed death (the cessation of sexual relations), raged at selfish, inconsiderate lovers, ached at the pain of sexual betrayal and rejection, and cried buckets of tears over a broken heart. I've learned along the way that it all goes with the erotic territory. And maybe my passionate personality.

The strangest thing about my life is that I never wanted to be controversial, notorious, or in the public eye—and somehow I have managed all three. I wanted to tell the truth, I wanted to expose lies, and in the beginning I naively thought this would make me seem courageous, maybe even honorable.

I started writing in the area of sexuality by accident. I was formerly a book reviewer, but always had an abiding interest and (seemingly) limitless curiosity about sexuality. When I read about other sexuality writers, we all seem to have this curiosity about sex, and we acknowledge that this is where people keep their deepest, darkest secrets. I had a desire to dig down and find out what people were hiding and why they were remaining hidden in their sexuality.

As a writer I have always lived by Dorothy Allison's belief that writers have to tell the truth; otherwise they are writing lies. I used to have that quote stuck above the desk where I wrote. I put it there to remind me to be courageous. I started writing from that vision for truth, that curiosity toward the women I knew, the women I had sex with, the gay men I hung out with, and the men I met through the sex industry.

So I started to write and research, and I found an eager market in the emerging gay publications. I developed regular readers whose support convinced editors to keep publishing my (then) off-the-wall views on sex and sexuality. When I was still considered too "controversial" for lesbian magazines, it was gay-male magazines that supported my work and allowed me to publish the first Australian articles on the feminist sex wars and the emerging lesbian SM scene.

Sometimes I still don't see what I did or wrote that was so outrageous, because I based my columns and articles about female sexuality and, specifically, about lesbian sexual culture on the stories of the women around me and on what I was doing with my lovers. I didn't make it up, although my detractors often accused me of making up sensational lies to either (a) advance my own career or (b) shock and disturb the equilibrium of the gay-girl world.

When I wrote about SM it was because we were doing it. When I wrote about discovering my femme identity, loving butches, and playing with gender, it was because I was doing it and so were the women around me. It came as a great shock, therefore, to be regularly pilloried because of my outrageous views, to have acquaintances refuse to acknowledge me in public lesbian venues, and to have editors nervously triple-checking my articles for something that might offend readers.

When I started writing about the sex industry it was as an insider. Like the other areas I explored, it was as a participant, not a voyeur. I believe that the weight of lies and the damage from stereotypes add another layer of oppression on women who make their living in the adult industry.

I see myself as a warrior with words, a sexual scribe. Words are my weapons and where the power of my influence lies. I've been writing since I could hold a pencil, and I cannot envisage a time when I will stop. But fifteen years down the track I am now doing a lot of reassessing. I took a ten-year journey through the SM world, but that world is now not where I choose to live. I will always be a femme, but not necessarily in relation to a butch. My sexual identity is much more fluid than before. I now don't want to expose my life, relationships, and friends in print; I feel the need for privacy and reflection more than candid exposure in the name of getting at the truth.

What still remains important is to speak up about political sexual repression.

Tips for Safer Sex in the World

✳ Write a letter to your local legislator today about a sexual issue in your district. Are the police harassing sex workers? Is your local adult shop under attack?

✳ At a dinner party bring up the topic of sexual rights and responsibilities and get people into a heated debate.

✳ Abortion is sexual freedom of choice. Point this out to friends and colleagues.

✳ Homophobia is sexual repression. Say so at every opportunity.

✳ Don't let anyone get away with jokes about sex workers or sexual violence toward women (so-called rape jokes). These are both based on sexual hatred.

✳ Do something sexually joyful for yourself every week— flirt with a stranger, wear something extra special and sexy to bed (no excuses just because you are sleeping alone), or think up a new potent sexual fantasy (don't just rely on the old ones).

✳ Remember the three Ms: massage, masturbation, and meditation. Make them a regular part of your life.

PART 5

Physical Challenges

In an era when discussion of sexuality is supposedly open and without limits, a significant number of women exists whose sexual issues fail to register on the agenda for discussion and whose sexuality is almost seen as taboo. These are women who are aging or facing physical challenges or ill health. In the late twentieth century, sexuality is portrayed as an activity for the beautiful, young, and physically "perfect." This is particularly reinforced in film, where the Hollywood erotic ideal and gymnastic sexuality dominate—standards few people can live up to even if they wanted to. In the celluloid world people are easily orgasmic and always satisfied, and "ugly" bodily fluids never spoil a beautiful erotic moment.

The perception of perfect bodies, perfect sex, and multiple orgasms excludes a large percentage of the human race whose sexuality is often complicated, less than satisfactory, or beset by physical and emotional contradictions. Perpetuating only a limited range of what is the acceptable face of sexuality leaves a large percentage of women who are postmenopausal, physically challenged, or living with a life-threatening illness with few places to go for an alternative view.

Although they are traditionally viewed as "sexless," these women often have a personal sexual expression that is a source of joy and physical delight. In their triumphant sexuality they defy Hollywood-imposed stereotypes, yet they are still not positively represented in public depictions of the sexually active.

Aging

Pregnancy was once viewed as a "sickness." Pregnant women were regarded as unsexual and unsexy and felt forced to hide their big bellies under tent-like maternity clothes. This view has changed as gutsy pregnant women rebelled and started to demand that they be seen as normal and healthy. When pregnant celebrities such as Demi Moore posed for nude photo spreads, the view of the pregnant body permanently altered.

The same revolution for postmenopausal women is yet to come. Menopause is only just coming off the "not to be discussed in public" list, but it is still viewed in many quarters as an illness rather than a normal, inevitable part of every woman's life. As the baby-boomer generation hits menopause this view is being transformed, and the same women who said, "Pregnancy is not an illness" are now saying "and neither is menopause."

However, images in popular culture do not reflect the shift, and older women still must struggle with outmoded stereotypes that equate female beauty with youthfulness. Consequently, older women remain disempowered and are viewed as less than beautiful. By contrast, in cultures where women's power and status are not tied to youthfulness, their value to society increases as they age.

Ancient cultures that revered the triple goddess—whose manifestations are maid, mother, and crone—gave equal value to each of these stages of every woman's life. When a woman reached her crone stage, she was seen as wise, with the knowledge of a lifetime at her fingertips. Her aging skin, white hair, and gnarled fingers were seen to have their own unique beauty. It is rare in Western culture today to see an older woman who looks like this described as beautiful, even rarer for her to be described as sexual.

Physical Challenges

The physically challenged have the same right as able-bodied people to a sexual expression they deem appropriate. Their situation often means they need an understanding caregiver who is able to act on their behalf—for example, purchasing sex toys or arranging for a sex surrogate. Caregivers themselves may fear that intervention on their clients' behalf could be misinterpreted as inappropriate sexual behavior, and so may be reluctant to advocate for their clients in this area. However, caregivers are frequently family members or a parent—and to negotiate the role of a sexually active adult with one's parent might be embarrassing.

While the traditional role of the church in running institutions and other facilities for the physically challenged has been beneficial, this solution has often been at the cost of ignoring the sexual needs and rights of these people. The problem arises not only from religious dogma or sexual intolerance; caregivers in such institutions may share the embarrassment of the wider community when confronted by the sexuality of people with disabilities.

Because it is difficult for people with disabilities to meet sexual partners, their ability to explore their own sexuality remains limited. Their opportunities for spontaneous sex might be restricted by the necessity to negotiate wheelchairs, catheters, or colostomy bags. The partners of physically challenged people need sensitivity and patience, and when both partners are physically challenged their intimate life may require the intervention of their caregivers.

A view of sexuality that says sex is for the physically perfect by definition excludes anyone who lives daily with muscle spasms, limited movement, or speech difficulties. Such a restricted view is ignorant and can cruelly affect the sexual self-esteem of people living with physical challenges.

Illness

Those who suffer from chronic or life-threatening illness often find ways to keep their sexuality alive. Many people facing serious illness see their sexuality as a connection to the life force. Yet, sick people are rarely seen as sexual; to view them this way is often regarded as obscene.

There is a way to strike a balance between looking after someone and still allowing him or her the dignity of sexual expression. While no one should be coerced into a sexual situation when ill, if someone requests intimate time with his or her partner, this should not be viewed as abhorrent.

Sexuality can manifest in lots of different ways besides heterosexual, penetrative sex. Erotic touch and massage can be a healing, affirmative expression of love and a healing moment for someone feeling disconnected from her or his body when dealing with illness. To be touched is to feel loved; this truth does not change from childhood until death. A massage service set up for people living with HIV/AIDS has reported wonderful feedback, even when clients have been in great pain or in the terminal stages of the disease.

In this part, the personal experiences of Joan Nestle and the work of Tuppy Owens and Rosie King illuminate the connections among the body, illness, aging, physical challenges, and being sexually alive.

Let My Desire Remain

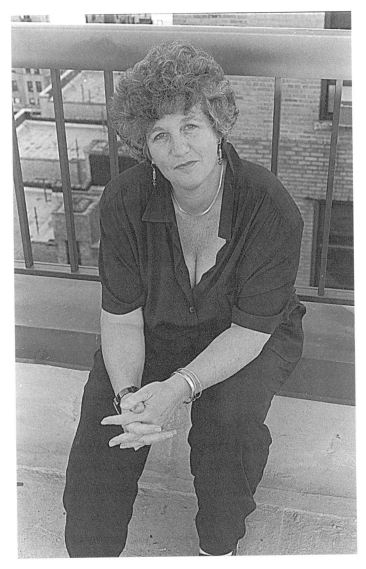

Kathryn Kirk

Joan Nestle was born in New York City in 1940, a working-class Jew raised by her mother, who worked as a bookkeeper in the garment industry. Joan came out as lesbian in Greenwich Village in the 1950s, marched in Selma in 1965,

*joined the ranks of the feminist movement in 1971, and helped establish the Gay
Academic Union in 1972. In 1973, Joan cofounded the Lesbian Herstory
Archives, which now fills a three-story building in Park Slope, Brooklyn.*

Joan is the author of A Restricted Country *and editor of* The Persis-
tent Desire: A Femme-Butch Reader. *She is coeditor (with Naomi
Holoch) of* Worlds Unspoken: An Anthology of International Lesbian
Fiction *and of the lesbian-fiction series* Women on Women. *With John Pre-
ston, she coedited* Sister and Brother: Lesbians and Gay Men Write
About Their Lives Together.

*She has won numerous awards, including the Bill Whitehead Award for
Lifetime Achievement in Lesbian and Gay Literature, the American Library
Association Gay/Lesbian Book Award, and the Lambda Literary Award for Les-
bian Nonfiction. She lives in New York.*

The following is an extract from Joan Nestle's book A Fragile Union
(San Francisco: Cleis Press, 1998).

15 January 1997

I haven't been able to write a word since I was told I have colon cancer. All of it—the bleeding, the tests, the operation, the chemo, the
fissure that will not heal, and the doctors who did everything so fast
and did not listen to me—all now embody everything I detest,
including my own body. Embody. I embody disease and disavowal,
blood and shit and a body bound in pain. Everything tastes like acid
now, like car batteries in my mouth. If ever words could bring me
life, and they have, please, please do it now.

The Ex-Lover

She stands, so fresh and open, in the doorway, a gray scarf hung
loosely from her muscled neck. Her green winter jacket is already
zipped, and in her right hand is a large blue carryall, bulging with
tools. I turn to say good-bye and all time stops. This woman with
whom I have shared a decade as lovers.

This woman who sat by my bed in a darkened hospital room,
hour after hour, keeping guard. One night in the hazy but impene-
trable sleep of drugs, I felt someone tug at my fingers and thought
it was the nurse taking my blood, but it was my love gently sliding

back onto my finger the ring she had given me ten years ago, before the flood of cells.

The Reading: February 1998

A year after my surgery, I was asked to participate in a reading from a new collection of lesbian erotica. The editor had selected my story "A Different Place," a story written in 1986 that celebrated the pleasure of anal fucking. This was my first public appearance as a writer since the cancer, and up to the last minute I did not know if I would be able to read that story in public. Everyone before me read from their piece that appeared in the collection. When I stepped up to the microphone, I thought I would give it a try, but as I read the opening passages of the story, describing the preparation Jay was going through to be ready to perform anal penetration, I knew that I would stop before the scene of entry.

I have colon-rectal cancer and it may kill me; that story over- whelmed the narrative of a night of pleasure in Connecticut over ten years ago. Torn between still wanting to preserve the space I had opened for my audience, the space that allowed women to enjoy all forms of sexual activity, and my own recent need for sexual silence, I chose as gracefully as I could to leave them with the sense of won- derful expectation, the promise that the story would bring them pleasure—but I could not go there with them, I explained, because of my cancer.

My Body

This is now my battle, to win back from the specifics of medical treatment—from the outrage of an invaded body where hands I did not know touched parts of myself that I will never see—my own body, my own body so marked by the hands and lips of lovers, now so lonely in its fear. Touch my scar, knead my belly, don't be afraid of my cancer. Enter me the old way, not through the skin cut open, but because I am calling to you through the movement of my hips, the breath that pleads for your hand to touch the want of me. Heal me because you do not fear me, touch me because you do not fear the future. Cancer and sex. One I have and one I must have.

The New Lover

Like a little girl bringing out a favorite doll, I shouted from the bedroom, "I need to show you something." You, my new friend, were sitting at the dining room table and turned expectantly toward me when I reappeared. "I need you to see this," I said, holding up my shirt and pulling down the band of my pants so you could see the still-red scar that started at my waist, skirted my belly button, and made its way down to the beginning of my pubic triangle.

I stood in front of you, not clear about why I was doing this, a fifty-seven-year-old woman exhibiting her cancer scar to a new friend. You reached out and traced the path of the incision with your fingers, and I started to cry. Not a little girl any more, but a woman with colon cancer, a cancer that should have been found when I had the colonoscopy done a year before the tumor grew so large it invaded the surrounding tissue, but that a rushed doctor had missed.

"I pulled out too quickly," he told me later, after the tumor had broken through the wall of my colon and spilled red blood into the toilet bowl. "Have you cried yet?" he asked me in 1997. It took a year for the tears to come, and they came only when I stood in front of a woman whom I wanted to touch me, to make love to me like it used to be.

My Treatment

It will never be like it used to be. Cancer has claimed me; "my cancer," I say now, like others talk about their cars or children. We suggest you have a year of chemo, the doctors said, and I did—or as much of it as I could stand. For that whole year, I did not allow anyone to touch me, except doctors, nurses, technicians. My body was filled with chemicals that sickened me. I sat on the edges of tables in small cubicles, the IV needle precariously housed in my arm, in a small vein on the back of my hand, or anywhere else the oncologist could find a vein large enough and strong enough to absorb the needle and the acid. Sometimes the vein would collapse, and the chemo would start pouring out under my skin. "You are lucky," the doctor said. "This chemo is not as dangerous as some of the others." And I knew he was right; I was one of the "lucky" ones. I would keep my hair; I avoided a shunt; I only had five hundred milligrams of 5-FU every week with fifty milligrams of Leucovorin, a form of folic acid, a natural substance that some people want to ingest. I had not been able to take the initial treatment, 5-FU with Ergamisole, a drug used to kill worms in the stomachs of sheep. After two treatments with the little white pills, I did not care if I lived or died.

This is not the story of every cancer patient; it is my own, just like this cancer, this colon-rectal cancer, is my own. Just like this body, now a year and a half after the surgeon removed four feet of colon, my transverse colon, and reattached my intestines in a new configuration, is my own. I need you to know all the details, the scientific names, the side effects, just as I had to learn them. Illness, like sex, gives the body another dimension, makes it transparent. I could feel the chemotherapy liquid enter my veins, trace its burning journey through my arm, just as I used to feel a lover's tongue trail down my neck.

Like so many others, I am caught in the limbo of cancer, the still place at the heart of the night. I cannot travel back to the physical safety I once thought I had, and I cannot go forward with any assurances that I have a future. I am not unique in this stasis, but this is my bedroom, my history; these are my questions of endurance. How will I travel in my life? What belongings will I carry with me? Let my desire remain, even if the cancer grows again into its gray mounds of life. Let my breasts and cunt grow hard with answering determination. And let me keep what I have learned from this illness—that terror is a human thing, that the body, even in its vomit and blood, wants to stand on its feet again, that kindness makes its way through the dead skin, that sickness, too, yearns for its human voice. These are my travels. Late in the night, I will go deep into my body's story and hear its tale of life battling life. And as I welcomed home my other beloved travelers, I will bury my head in the gift of hope only I can bring to the surface.

A Healthy Sex Life for All

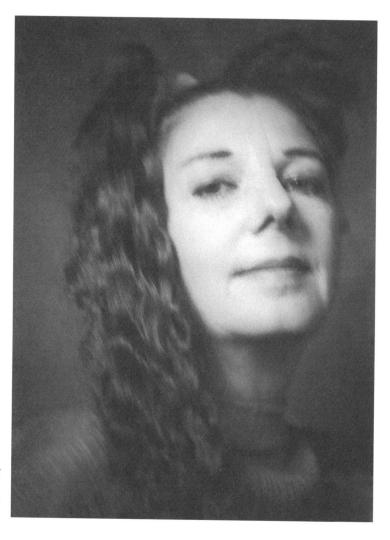

Aiden Kelly

Tuppy Owens has a diploma in human sexuality from London University and an honorary doctorate for her "good works." Born in Cambridge, U.K., she was the second child of a university-educated man from a well-to-do background and a local girl from a working-class family. Her father was known for his dirty jokes, so she grew up learning that sex was funny. While her father let her do as she wanted, when her mother discovered a letter Tuppy had written about trying to have sex with a man, Tuppy was ordered straight off to Sunday school.

When she was seventeen, Tuppy traveled to the Serengeti to join her boyfriend counting wildebeest. When she returned to London she studied zoology at Exeter, whizzed away to Trinidad, and eventually ended up back in London, where she discovered pornography on her boyfriend's father's printing press. It was to change her life.

✳✳✳

I felt that existing pornographic magazines were an insult to sex, so I rushed out to take some better photos and design better books. I was amazed when told that the self-portraits I'd taken on a river-bank at dawn with a doll up me were illegal. I accepted the restrictions and went on to produce a very happy book that stayed within the law, titled *Sexual Harmony*. It included pretty photos of a charming couple in lots of exciting sex positions as well as my attempts to explain how to fuck and have fun.

What I had done for free as a challenge became a nice little money earner; the books sold a hundred copies a week in a new London sex shop. This financed other photo shoots, and soon I was producing a series, *Love in the Open Air*, with pics taken in the British countryside of couples copulating, in spring, summer, autumn, and winter. My writing gained confidence and became quite tender and poetic.

One Christmas, a gay couple from Amsterdam visited me and on departing promised to send me a saucy Dutch diary as a thank-you gift. Halfway into January, it still hadn't arrived (there was probably no such thing) and I began to fantasize about turning the pages of a dated scrapbook to discover a lovely porno pic in front of my eyes every morning of the year. The idea grew, and I decided to produce a *Sex Maniac's Diary* to mimic the other hobbyist diaries of the era, one giving facts and figures, all presented formally. As well as its being a great joke, I liked the idea of treating sex with the same respect and detail as other pastimes.

The 1973 *Sex Maniac's Diary* came out on 12 December 1972 and sold out in two weeks. I continued producing this little book for twenty-three years. At its peak, it was selling over one hundred thousand copies a year. The *Diary* gave me the chance to research what was going on in the swing and fetish scenes and many other scenes all over the world, so I became something of an international expert. Clubs and hotels were reviewed but were also allocated symbols, denoting certain erotic characteristics and qualities. When AIDS hit, I reviewed condoms and drew pictures from Polaroids I'd shot of me and my then-favorite cock of how to put on a condom. I changed the name to the *Safer Sex Maniac's Diary*.

I took great pride in the project and worked very hard to produce each issue. By the time the *Diary* was established, I had made friends with Annie Sprinkle and a few other pioneers around the world, and we took pleasure in each other's existence. Distributors often tried to censor the *Diary*, as I listed very extreme clubs and groups, but I always found a way to carry on, continuing to include the bizarre things simply by using language the distributors wouldn't understand. I eventually compiled a book called *Planet Sex: The Handbook*, with loads of info in it, and dumped the *Diary* for good in 1995.

Producing one annual a year gave me some spare time. In 1978 I met a couple of disabled people who had no social or sexual lives. I helped them remedy their situation and thought there must be lots of other isolated people who, with a little reassurance and a few introductions, could have their lives transformed. With a healthy sex life, the disability, pain, and disfigurement might even feel less troublesome.

I started Outsiders in 1979 as a dating club for people with disabilities. It was run from my home, and after a couple of newspaper articles we got lots of fabulous members and held parties, lunches, and discussions. We compiled a book called *Practical Suggestions*, published a list of members and a magazine, and it was all tremendous fun. Then the residents of my block objected to my working from home, and I was faced with having to rent an office. So I began the Sex Maniac's Ball to raise funds.

Outsiders now has a bright, wheelchair-accessible office in Holland Park, is run by a small band of loyal disabled members, has a management committee of members with varied disabilities, and is moving from strength to strength. This isn't to say we haven't had problems. These have come mostly from the more radical disabled world, where they see self-help groups for disabled people run by so-called able-bodied people—let alone by someone involved in pornography—as suspect. Little did they know that just before I began Outsiders, I'd broken up with a boyfriend and found myself totally isolated and suffering panic attacks. So more than just acting as a philanthropy-minded able-bodied porn aficionado, I could actually relate from my own experiences to the feelings of loneliness and frustration endured by members of Outsiders.

Being a woman sex writer and a self-employed publisher, especially in the field of sex, was isolating. The club also got attacked by the gutter press, which made up a story linking whores and disability. We have never really recovered. Some members told me that before coming to an Outsiders event, people in their residential homes teased them about their forthcoming orgy—a painful experience if you're still a virgin and desperate to find a loving partner.

Even today, some radical disability activists say that any relationship between a disabled person and an able-bodied person must be exploitative. I know differently. One of our first couplings was between a girl with mild learning difficulties and a chemistry teacher with acne. Very happy they were too. I remember a blind girl asking her father what he thought of her new boyfriend, and Dad complained that he was black—which was news to the blind girl— but she didn't care! We accept everyone for who and what they are, so long as they don't express prejudice of any kind. We acknowledge their sexuality, however disabled or disfigured they might be. I wish we had more success, but doesn't everyone wish for more of that! We always have too many men and not enough women. Women are put off by our sexy reputation and are often incredibly timid. On top of that, it's easier for disabled women to find partners in a society where men want someone to have sex with and to marry, and women feel they should have a partner their parents and friends will approve of.

Many of the men complain bitterly of sexual frustration; few of the women do. We've had to be careful about introducing men to prostitutes, because we could get busted for pimping. In any case, most prostitutes don't use their time with the men to educate and teach them, they just provide an easy (and enjoyable) screw or fantasy experience that does little to help the chap go out and find a real relationship. I'd like to train surrogates, but that will have to wait until our laws are reformed.

Soon after I started Outsiders, I decided to take a course in sex therapy and was delighted to get into a two-year postdoctorate course at a London hospital as part of London University. This gave me loads of confidence and the capacity to answer the questions of members of Outsiders with more knowledge. I got invited to talk about the club at conferences; it seemed that people in foreign countries were far more impressed. Back home, people still preferred to attack me.

While I was touring America doing research for the *Sex Maniac's Diary*, I was meeting dozens of really interesting sexual adventurers who were running clubs and doing other things, but none of them ever met each other. I decided to put on an international erotic event and realized it could also raise funds for Outsiders. I felt rather like Robin Hood: using those who have plenty to provide for those who have none. The first Sex Maniac's Ball was held in 1986, and it was wild. I had no idea how to run a club or a large party, but over a thousand people from all over the world showed up. We definitely were not invited back to that venue (the London Dungeon)! I am about to embark on planning the fourteenth annual event, and once again I have yet to find a venue.

I encourage disabled people to come, as well as swingers, fetishists, and boogiers. But most of all, I encourage people to attend who have minority tastes and have never expressed them in public, so they can be "out" and others can meet and accept them. Most of the resulting sideshows and spectacles raise a bit of cash for Outsiders, besides providing fun and entertainment. Keeping all these revelers responsibly in charge of their collection boxes is a job and a half! The ball has kept going during the entire rise and fall of the fetish scene in London, through the swelling popularity of swing clubs as swingers get used to condoms, and throughout youths' fascination with experimentation. I have to keep my eye on the moment and create a ball each year that will attract people despite the ebb and flow of fashion and trend. Having visited so many sex clubs around the world, I had a wealth of creativity to inspire me and get me started. We have a fabulous Grope Box, based on an idea I discovered at the swing club Sea Breeze in Marina del Rey, California. Thank you, Tom! I have yet to re-create your fabulous Infinity Room, lined with millions of tiny mirrors.

One of my inventions is the Rubber Wall—a large sheet of translucent backlit rubber, which you can dance or gyrate against and enjoy unknown bodies on the other side. The last ball had a Spanish theme to make everyone feel up and happy, and a troupe of girls did a flamenco dance on top of a fetishist who likes being trampled. Olé! Five years ago, I decided that there's not enough acclaim for people who rebel or excel in the sex industry and the erotic world. So I started the Erotic Oscars. This has been a really hard job. A fabulous team of judges decides nominations, finalists, and actual winners of the twelve categories, which include sex worker, filmmaker, and innovator. We put on a stunning exhibition, and the finalists who are performers do a show at the ball. One of the reasons for doing the Oscars is to give the winners positive publicity, but guess what? The press always ignores us. It's odd, isn't it? Magazines, newspapers, and TV are chock-a-block with sex, but they still want to portray the seamy side and ignore the innovators and the people who are really doing good things. Last year, we had the Oscars filmed by the BBC, so perhaps we'll get a higher profile in the future.

By the tenth anniversary of the Sex Maniac's Ball, I was beginning to feel confident that it would be socially acceptable. I booked a prestigious venue, designed a really exotic and rude flier, had loads of new ideas, and was ready for a big splash. Perhaps it had something to do with the British government's finally making anal sex legal and the fact that therefore on the flier I'd called the venue the Anal Academy, or perhaps we were too high profile, but the cops decided to stop the event. So fifteen hundred people, some of whom had flown in from as far away as Tokyo, arrived at an empty building, while I was trying to give the thousands of dollars worth of food prepared for the guests to London's homeless. I'd had so many setbacks before in my life that I took it all in stride.

Outsiders was broke, but we had been broke before. Still, other people were not amused, and after a public meeting, a march to the prime minister was organized and the Sexual Freedom Coalition was launched. The coalition is a pansexual, nonpartisan campaign for the sexual freedom of all consenting adults. It is concerned with law reform, responsible reporting of sex in the media, and educating and encouraging people to enjoy their sexuality to the full. I edit the campaign newspaper, *Consenting Adults*.

Tips for Physically Challenged People

The Outsiders have produced a book, *Practical Suggestions*, which lists pointers that have helped physically challenged people to date, chat, seduce someone, and have sex. We believe that physically challenged people are sexual, and the only way your friends will agree is if you talk about sex, expressing your frustrations and requesting help if you need it.

* Masturbate if you don't have a partner, and if you can't, tell someone and everyone about your need. A sex angel just might come along to do it for you.

* Don't allow people to fob you off with the notion that masturbation is enough. Everyone wants intimacy, and you need it just as much as the next person.

* Don't be sexually timid. You only live once. Take risks that might get you rejected; you may be pleasantly surprised. Otherwise you can go home and have a laugh with your friends.

* If people pity you, then pity them, for they don't know you very well and haven't bothered to discover how great you are.

* A dear friend of mine told me that physically challenged people make the best lovers because they have to think and plan the experience. Spread the word.

The Right Conditions for Lovemaking

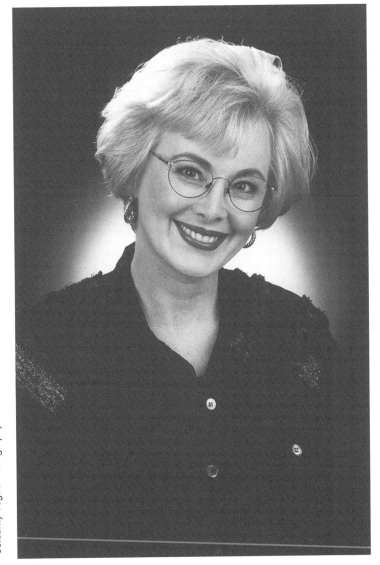

Celebrity Vogue Photography

Rosie King is a doctor with a difference. A sex therapist and sex educator, she has worked consistently in the Australian media for over a decade. Her weekly column in Woman's Day *and regular appearances on television's* The Midday Show *have helped to bring her warmth, humor, and sound advice into millions of Australian homes. She is a highly respected regular contributor to the newspaper the* Australian.

Rosie trained as a medical practitioner at the University of New South Wales and spent ten years in general practice. She is an honorary Fellow of the Australasian College of Sexual Health Physicians and a visiting lecturer at the University of New South Wales in the School of Obstetrics and Gynecology. She also lectures for the master of medicine and master of public health degrees at the University of Sydney. She is the author of a best-selling book, Good Loving, Great Sex.

✳✳✳

Having worked in the area of sexuality for many years, I recognize that I have the same fears, anxieties, and worries as everyone else. The fact that I recognize that I am not immune to these has given me a natural kindness when I work in this area. *Kindness* in this sense means that I feel "of a kind," part of the herd; I feel a sense of belonging. This reduces my sense of isolation and stops a feeling of disconnection, because I realize that we all have the same anxieties and worries.

When I was younger I used to think that the people who seemed very emotionally "together" didn't have any problems, whereas I spent all my time focusing on solving my problems. Eventually, however, I developed Rosie's Theory, which says that no matter how much time I spent trying to solve my problems there were always more to take their place. I decided that life contains a constant stream of problems, and although it is a good idea to problem-solve it cannot be the focus of living.

Since this realization, I have begun focusing on making sure there are more "goodies" in my life. My theory says that one goodie equals a hundred problems, and that happiness comes not from solving problems but from finding goodies. For me, goodies include having sex, walking my dogs, listening to music, spending time with my children, sleeping, and eating.

The key to happiness is not being problem-free. It is dealing with your problems and making sure there are lots of goodies in your life. That is where sex fits in. Sadly, for many people, sex is a source of disappointment, despair, frustration, anxiety, and pain. I keep working in this area because I would like sex to be a goodie for everyone.

Every day I accept and value my own sexuality more. I believe if ever you want proof that there is a God, you only have to look at the beauty of our sexuality to be convinced, because it is so perfect. I never get sick of talking, learning, thinking, and working about sex because I believe our sexuality is a miracle. Desire waxes and wanes naturally throughout life, but you don't need desire to enjoy sex.

Desire is affected by hormonal problems, physical illness, relationship difficulties, and the stresses of everyday life. However, given the right conditions, it is possible to become aroused and enjoy sex without any desire at all. Desire and arousal are two separate components and are run by different parts of the brain. Of course, it is much easier to be turned on if you start with a high level of desire. But even if initially you feel sexually uninterested, if your partner helps to warm you up then often you can enjoy a very pleasurable sexual experience, which can lead to high levels of arousal and orgasm.

There are many times when women feel sexual but don't feel like penetrative intercourse. At such times they might be quite happy to participate in sexual activity that is less demanding. It is important to realize that this is part of the give-and-take of a long-term relationship. Often partners need to negotiate a compromise; for example, in a heterosexual relationship he might have a need for sex and she may need to be sexually inactive. In such cases a couple can experience physical and emotional closeness without engaging in penetrative sex. This is where "outercourse" comes in very handy. It can expand your concept of lovemaking so that you can make love to your partner without necessarily getting turned on.

Desire is not the only reason for sex. Sex also encompasses the expression of love and affection, fun, pleasure given and received, passion, sensuality, communication, intimacy, procreation, sexual release, tension release, affirmation of desirability, security, confirmation of the relationship, affirmation of gender, nurturing, comfort, the inducing of sleep, pleasing one's partner, and the quenching of "skin hunger." Skin hunger, rather than sex drive, is the greatest motivator for sexual contact. A lot of casual sex is motivated by the need to be touched; it is a basic human need present from the time we are born. In the early twentieth century, studies were conducted in an orphanage comparing different levels of contact. Babies were separated into two groups: babies in one group were fed, bathed, and put back to bed, while babies in the other group were also cuddled. Infants in the group that received minimal touch became sick more often, failed to thrive, and had a higher mortality rate. The need to be touched doesn't stop because we reach puberty or age fifty; it remains an important part of being human. We are herd animals, like dogs or horses, and need skin-on-skin contact and touching for good general health.

To continue to make love throughout life, we have to ask ourselves what lovemaking is. Is it penis-vagina intercourse? For gay people that is not what sex is; they are much more flexible in their concept of sex. Lovemaking is a physical and emotional connection between two people, and it need not include desire, arousal, erection, lubrication, orgasm, or ejaculation. To express our sexuality to the fullest, we must let go of rigid ideas about what constitutes lovemaking. There are many people who, for all sorts of reasons, can't or don't have sexual intercourse.

Some branches of the Judeo-Christian tradition hold that sex is only for reproduction; this rules out all variations except penetrative sex, and I believe we are far beyond such a limited definition. There is a difference between making love and copulation. Copulation is for reproduction, while lovemaking involves a much higher spiritual, emotional, and physical connection. Sex is more than simply passing sperm to eggs.

We should be careful to avoid laying down guidelines of sexual behavior for women at certain times of life, such as after childbirth, menopause, or illness. These are common times for sexual desire to decrease in intensity. Interestingly, humans are the only animals that mate when the females are pregnant or after menopause.

Every woman is an individual, and it is true that some women feel less sexual around childbirth and in the early months of child rearing. It also might be that society doesn't see pregnant women as sexual beings—women are either "mothers" or "whores," not both. For some women it can take years for their sexual response to return. Some women feel sexy no matter what happens in their life, while for others their sexuality waxes and wanes. In our culture there has always been a bit of shame associated with pregnancy, with the pregnant body hidden behind voluminous maternity clothes. Western society tends to desexualize pregnant women, which is fine for some women, but not for others who feel very alive and sexual. One patient told me that during her pregnancy she felt like an earth goddess, the fountain of all living things.

Ill women certainly aren't seen as sexy. When someone assumes the role of patient, they become stripped of their identity, power, and status. Patients are often treated patronizingly, which leads to the person feeling disempowered and asexual. The patient becomes "the breast cancer in bed 24" or "the hysterectomy in bed 22." Sex is a very unwelcome visitor in hospitals; a doctor will discharge a patient with an A-to-Z list of dos and don'ts but often will fail to include an S for sexuality. This attitude needs to be updated. Research on cancer patients in the 1980s showed that even though sexual activity decreased after the cancer diagnosis, the level of intimacy and the need for touch and emotional connectedness grew more important.

Our society excludes the disabled and the ill from the fantasy model of sex. To enjoy sex when you have an illness, conditions need to be optimum, so you need to be sexually flexible. Intercourse may not be possible, so you may need to explore outercourse. Partners who are caregivers also need to be aware that changes occur in the dynamics of the relationship. The caregiver becomes more like a parent and the patient more like a child. If you wait for sex to happen spontaneously in this situation, often it won't. So there needs to be a deliberate space made for the sexual relationship. Once the caregiver has given attention or medication to the partner, it is a good idea to take a break from one another. Take a shower, change clothing, and meet each other as adult to adult, lover to lover, rather than caregiver-parent to patient-child.

When one partner is facing a serious or terminal illness, the well partner may try to protect himself or herself from the anticipation of pain and loss by distancing himself or herself from the sick partner. One partner may feel a need to be really close, while the other partner may deal with his or her grief by creating emotional distance. When Joy Davidman, wife of English author C. S. Lewis, was dying of bone cancer, she said, "The pain, then, is part of the pleasure now." She meant that if you really love somebody, there is always pain in the risk of losing them. Which would you rather do? Forgo the love and avoid the pain, or experience the love and accept that the pain is simply part of loving someone dearly? David Smarsh, who wrote *The Sexual Crucible*, said, "It takes tremendous courage to love right up to the moment of death."

People going through a transition from illness to health need to recognize that a grief process is necessary in the face of any loss. The loss may be tangible or intangible. Tangible losses are the alterations in body image: amputation, hair loss, radiation scarring, surgical scarring, tracheotomy, colonoscopy, changes in sexual functioning. What may have been possible before may no longer be possible. People need space to grieve those losses.

The intangible loss is of the fantasy future. In our own minds we often have a script about how things are going to be, and illness can disrupt this fantasy future. We need to grieve for it even though it is intangible, and then we need to create a new fantasy future. We need to rewrite our life script to incorporate illness or disability in a way that enhances rather than diminishes us.

People who are physically disabled typically don't fit into normal ideals of what is beautiful, and their sexual development and expression are very much moderated by the attitudes of society and their caretakers. Rehab programs exist for most areas of life function, but sexuality is usually ignored because disabled people don't fit into the stereotype of a sexually active person. Society has a tendency to assume that everyone in a wheelchair is the same, or everyone with a developmental delay is the same, when in fact people with so-called disabilities are just as individual as other members of the human race. Like everyone else, they have differences in potential for sexual expression, joy, and sharing. As health-care professionals practicing holistic care, we must look after the sexual needs of our patients as well as their physical, emotional, and intellectual needs.

Menopause is a state of hormone reduction that can affect cognitive functions, sometimes resulting in problems with memory, concentration, and decision making. These conditions can be extremely distressing. Muscle strength and durability are affected by the drop in testosterone levels, with a resultant muscular fatigue. Hormone replacement therapy (HRT) can be extremely helpful in reducing the incidence of heart disease, preventing osteoporosis, and improving general well-being. When a woman's estrogen levels drop, her skin's sensitivity decreases, her sense of smell decreases, her pheromone levels decrease—and all this can reduce her sense of sexuality. She feels like she has swapped the scent of a woman for the scent of a grandmother. Undergoing HRT can restore these very important functions.

For decades menopausal women were given estrogen and progestogen as hormone replacement. While they enjoyed physical and emotional benefits from this regimen, they didn't receive benefit in the area of sexual desire. When the ovaries stop producing estrogen and progestogen, there is also a reduction in testosterone levels, which bears a significant effect on female sex drive. Estrogen and progestogen replacement has a beneficial effect on sexual *response*, but not on sexual *drive*. It actually lowers any levels of testosterone remaining in the body; consequently, a woman may find that HRT means the end of her sex drive. Now, physicians also prescribe testosterone replacement to help with the sex drive.

For many women, however, menopause is the excuse they've been looking for to give up a sex life they never found rewarding. Other women are quite happy to accept the changes and to alter their sexual activity to encompass them, and still others say they enjoy sex more after menopause because they are free of the risk of pregnancy.

But menopause is not just a hormonal change; it is usually accompanied by many other changes in life. Often it involves a change of identity brought about by an empty nest and a shift in the primary relationship. As children leave home, the role of coparenting is lost. Or a woman may still have older, dependent children at home. It's a time involving changes for men, too, such as retrenchment, depression, alcohol problems, or sexual difficulties. Many start taking medication for the first time. And women in our society are not valued as sexual after reaching menopause. As Joanne Woodward said of her husband, Paul Newman, "He gets prettier and I get older."

Aging in our culture proves much more challenging for women than for men because it signals the end of women's reproductive capacity, whereas men maintain their reproductive capacity until death. Additionally, in Western society men are valued for what they do and what they have, and as their power and status increase (often with age), they are viewed as more sexually attractive. Women are valued by how they look, so when the characteristics regarded as "sexy" in a woman—such as smooth skin, a slim body, and firm breasts—decline, often so do their feelings of sexual attractiveness. Our visual media perpetuate these stereotypes. Sean Connery is considered very sexy, while Angela Lansbury is a "granny." Films depict older men with younger women, but you don't see it the other way around. The alternative is plastic surgery, creating women who look artificially age-free, such as Priscilla Presley, Raquel Welch, and Jane Fonda. These women are admired for remaining eternally youthful, making aging more and more a taboo for women.

Coping with the physical consequences of aging, even for people who enjoy good health overall, can seem like fighting an uphill battle. So instead of obsessing about "losing your looks," why not focus on developing the inner qualities of self-confidence, a sense of humor, serenity, and a vibrant spirit? These gifts will make you less susceptible to the depression and loss of self-esteem that otherwise can accompany the inevitable failings of the flesh that come with aging. And don't forget that maturing, after all, is part of the plan of Mother Nature.

Exercise: Finding Your Own Right Conditions for Sex

Given the right conditions, sexual arousal is possible. Burnie Zilbergeld, author of *Men and Sex*, offers an exercise to help discover what those conditions are for you.

* Think of your three best sexual experiences. If you can't remember any, imagine what one would be like. Now write down all the conditions that made the experiences good. They could include privacy, having plenty of time, an exciting atmosphere, an adventurous sexual activity, a comfortable place, being with someone you love, or feeling good about your body.

* Next, recall your three worst sexual experiences. Again, use your imagination if you've been lucky enough never

to have had a negative sexual experience. Now write down the conditions that made the experiences negative. These might include tension, being rushed, feeling pressured, feeling afraid, being physically uncomfortable, feeling violated, not speaking up about your desires, having other worries and stresses on your mind.

✳ What you now have is a list of your own positive and negative conditions for sex. The idea is to be aware of these so you can begin to consciously maximize and increase the positive conditions and recognize and minimize the negative ones. While we may wish or believe that feeling sexual "just happens," in truth, a good sexual experience requires proactive participation. Learning to minimize the negative and maximize the positive is a gradual process, so don't forget to be patient with yourself and your partner(s).

PART 6

Domination and Submission

Surveys of people's sexual fantasies are always fascinating. One of the most interesting aspects of these peeks into the fantasy realm is to see how fantasies differ according to age, gender, or sexual preference. Just as fascinating is how these indicators sometimes make no difference at all in the type of fantasies people have. And the number-one area where this is the case is domination and submission, where fantasies of being overpowered show up strongly and consistently. It seems that most of us, at least some of the time, fantasize of being dominated and forced into sex. For many, this also involves physical discipline of some sort, from having our bottoms playfully spanked to being severely whipped.

Most people do not act on these fantasies, content to leave them in an imaginary erotic world. For those who do, the results can be profound. Many report that this type of sexual adventure has reignited their relationship's sexual flame. It can reintroduce excitement into a relationship that has been bogged down in the familiar. To create good SM (sadomasochism) play requires planning, building anticipation, and a dramatic flair, and this level of communication and forward planning is great for any couple's sexuality.

Some people go further and decide to permanently incorporate aspects of dominant and submissive roles into not only their sexual expression, but their daily lives. These couples take on an SM lifestyle that is physically intense and often includes an unexpected spiritual dimension. The deep love between an SM couple, which often seems to break all the rules on what makes a good relationship, can be a shock to other people.

For people wanting to get into SM but with no way to access the scene, a visit to a professional dominatrix is a great first step.

This gives a safe, professional introduction to the scene and a way to learn SM etiquette, how to set limits, discuss fantasies, and be introduced to the range of dominant-submissive erotic possibilities. Alternatively, if a private SM organization or social club exists in your area, attending one of its events would be a good way to learn safety and socializing techniques. It is important to get support, because amateurs can often make mistakes.

One of the hardest things SM players must deal with is the widespread misunderstanding about SM from those outside the scene. People who know nothing of the structure of SM play often erroneously view SM as nonconsensual and abusive (or potentially abusive). SM play is always consensual and fully negotiated; activities are agreed to ahead of time. SM players do this to minimize risks to each other's physical and emotional well-being, and to make sure that all parties get what they want from the interaction: erotic pleasure and/or personal growth.

Often, people get scared by SM paraphernalia—leather, rubber, studs, and whips and chains. For others, these are just the outward manifestation of the domination and submission that turns them on. Yet, while these props and this look can reinforce domination, they alone do not make a dominant a convincing wielder of power. That quality comes from within.

Domination and submission play can cover everything from teasingly making someone your sex "slave" for an hour to a long, severely painful session of discipline and sexual torture. Bondage and discipline (BD) is the most well-known side of SM, but it is only one part of its rich tapestry. Nevertheless, it is the aspect most people are familiar with and the one most subject to nudge-nudge sexual jokes and innuendoes.

Below, I offer some definitions:

Top: the dominant partner in dominant-submissive play.

Bottom: the submissive partner in dominant-submissive play.

Switch: someone who can play either the dominant or submissive role in sexual play; also refers to a dominant-submissive play session in which players change roles halfway through.

Play: participating in an SM scene; it is called this because participants are actually playacting a fantasy role. It is an extension of the childhood game of dress-up.

Fetish: when sexual feelings are triggered by objects, parts of the body, certain clothes, or types of materials. The most well-known material fetishes are fur, leather, and rubber. A fetishism for shoes or boots is the most common clothing fetish. A fetish can be mild or extreme; in extreme cases the material or object is essential to sexual arousal.

✳✳✳

For most people and couples, SM begins and ends in their own private space or in a discreet SM environment. Some women who are involved in the scene in their personal lives eventually make a career out of their natural dominant talents and work as professional mistresses. Likewise, there are many women who work professionally as mistresses who have no personal interest in SM in their private lives.

In this part, Kat Sunlove, Cléo Dubois, and Amanda Dwyer share decades of their own experience in the roles of erotic domination and submission and their tips on how to re-create this fantasy at home.

The Desire to Be Helpless and the Wish to Wield Power

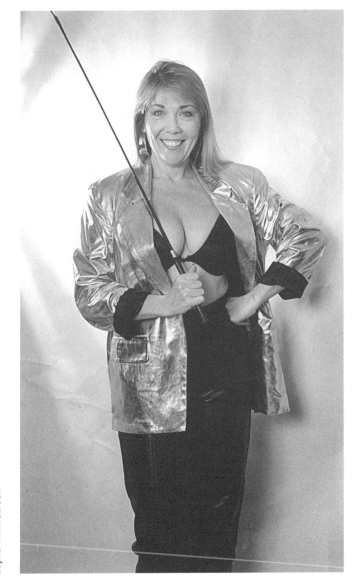

Layne Winklebleck

Since the early 1980s Kat Sunlove has been involved in the sex industry as a performer, journalist, educator, publisher of Spectator, *and since late 1997 as a lobbyist for the Free Speech Coalition. With a masters in political science, a year of law school, and many years of political activism, Kat is well suited for the challenges of advocating for the interests of the sex industry. She lives in Sacramento, California, but her activism spreads across the United States.*

Better known as Mistress Kat to her submissive fans, Kat wrote a weekly advice column on erotic dominance and submission for four years in the early 1980s in Spectator *and later for the national magazine* Chic; *these activities earned her the label of the Dear Abby of SM. With her life partner, Layne Winkleback, she designed and taught a popular workshop series titled* SM for Loving Couples, *the first serious educational workshops on this sensational and misunderstood topic. The workshops were featured in an anthropological study of the San Francisco SM community,* Erotic Power, *by Dr. Gini Graham Scott.*

Kat and Layne have been guest lecturers at San Francisco State University, University of the Pacific, and the Institute for the Advanced Study of Human Sexuality. They have appeared on numerous radio and television programs dealing with erotic fantasy play, censorship, and sexual freedom. For several years the couple worked to produce a major theatrical production starring Mistress Kat on the theme of erotic female dominance.

Kat was a contributor to the original Cyborgasm *CD project, now distributed through Time-Warner. She was the inspiration for the first radical sex photo book by Michael Rosen,* Sexual Magic: The S/M Photographs. *In 1995 Kat produced and starred in her own Fabulous at Fifty Fantasy Ball to celebrate her birthday as well as to promote the idea of the sexiness of older women.*

She is a member of Feminists for Free Expression, NOW, COYOTE, the San Francisco Press Club, and the Society of Professional Journalists, and she was a founder of the anticensorship group Cal-ACT. She now serves as the Executive Director of National ACT.

✳✳✳

For some years in the early 1980s my life partner, Layne Winklebleck, and I conducted what we've been told were the first-ever serious workshops on erotic dominance and submission, or SM. Inspired by our own very self-conscious erotic adventures in this mysterious world of power, we felt that we could help other loving couples bypass some of the pitfalls of such an intimate exploration of the darker side of our psyches. It is, after all, a scary place to go:

the desire to be helpless, to be taken, to be swept away by another's desire. Or conversely, the wish to inflict pain or to wield power over another for one's own selfish sexual gratification. Or so it all appears to the uninitiated. In fact, it's much more complex than that and much more profound.

As Layne and I began playing with power in our own lovemak-
ing, I was struck by the intense erotic thrill I got from his dominant attentions. At that point in my life, age thirty-four, I was identifying as a lesbian, having found men to be too much work. But Layne, a longtime friend, was different. I trusted him and had lusted after him; I knew the quality of his character. So when he put his hand on my throat during sex, I relaxed and enjoyed the delicious sensations that coursed through my body.

Afterwards, I questioned him endlessly, trying to understand what could be so exciting about submitting to a man when I felt that submission to men was largely what had gotten women into the second-class mess we were in. His communication skills and understanding of the human mind, honed by years as a therapist and as a teacher of graduate students in social work, enabled him to gently lead me into a deeper and deeper exploration of these amazing ener-
gies. Almost in spite of myself, I was drawn into the taboo world of power play. The experiences were telepathic. We would each feel a dark thrill—a growling, blood-thickening rush, we called it—when our respective mental and emotional states were tuned into each other like some errant radio wave that finally finds the right channel. He, the lustful, harsh master; I, the willing, accepting slave.

And still, as much as I came to enjoy and appreciate my submis-
sive side, I could not fathom wanting to hurt him or to dominate him. But I was curious. He suggested that I try slapping him during a lovemaking session one night when I was atop him. I gave his face a light blow, and we laughed at my reticence. Then he said, "Go ahead, try again. I'll still love you even if you hurt me." Unable to resist the challenge, I let go and slapped him full-out. The rush I felt was frightening to me, so strongly did it throb in my cunt. By pushing past my own limits, I had discovered my sadistic potential. But I was afraid of it, fearful that I would actually hurt someone to feel that thrill.

By continuing our explorations, both together and with others, however, I learned that I would not hurt anyone. I merely seek out those who would enjoy and revel in the other side of that erotic dyad. We also learned that there are some emotional risks in this kind of play. You must know and trust your partner. And your partner must be trustworthy. Safe words don't matter to a psychopath, so you have to be sure that the person you choose to play with is sane. The submissive must be able ultimately to take care of their own needs, to ask for love and gentleness when the dominant forgets to show affection. The dominant must always remember it's a game intended for pleasure, and they must not slip over the edge from pushing limits to violating them.

Eventually, I turned the tables on Layne and became the dominant of his dreams, and he became the submissive of dreams I never really knew I had. We threw ourselves into a pursuit of knowledge and experience of this misunderstood area of human sexuality. For almost a year, we read everything we could find on the subject (not much). We even experimented with lifestyle dominance and submission, but eventually we found that it was not for us.

We decided that the oppression both sexes feel in modern society is role-based, not gender-based. In other words, the dominant, whether male or female, gets tired of always making the decisions, initiating the action, taking care of the bottom. Similarly, the submissive may begin to feel unappreciated, underloved, or misused by the top. Both can feel taken for granted if there is not enough "straight time," time to be real and talk about one's feelings, about what is working for each and what is not. Communication in this arena, just as in many other parts of life, is the key. People who are not honest with themselves or who do not know themselves well and who do not listen to their partner are often unable to achieve the personal growth and erotic satisfaction available through SM play. They can get lost in their own fantasies and mistake submission for stupidity, dominance for callousness.

In our workshops, we focused on female dominance and male submission, not because of an erotic bias, but rather because that had been the direction of our greatest learning and because we felt that was the direction most likely to benefit society. To help a man get in touch with his desire for submission, to allow a woman room to explore her dominant fantasies seemed likely to help both. To get a woman in touch with her own erotic power and with the ability to use that power lovingly with a partner, to help her understand why he wants and needs the experience of submission—these were our motivations in designing the workshops.

Our messages were simple. To the women we said, "Find your own dominant style; explore your own fantasies. Listen to his fantasies but only as fuel for your own. Use what you like and stay true to your own energy. Plan ahead. Tease, tease, tease. Create a fantasy world of your own in which you can have your sexual desires fulfilled. Play safe. Try the equipment on yourself so you know what you are doing to his body. A crop hurts far more than a flogger, despite their relative appearance. Stay sane. Go far enough to 'scratch his itch' but not so far as to really do harm. Hypnotize him with voice, eyes, touch. Tune into him and follow the energy. Show him your love and your magnificence as well as your dominance." To the men we said, "Let go of your fantasized wants and let her use you for her desires. Be genuine in your submission. Love her dominant self. Respect her. Let yourself be taken. Be patient as she learns the ropes. Never leave egg on her face by telling her she isn't doing it right. Don't be so goal-orientated. Enjoy the flow of energy. Open up and let her see your soft side. Relax, relax, and breathe." We didn't encourage so-called safe words. Instead, we put the dominant in charge and made her fully responsible for staying in control of safety as well as sex. We did encourage straight time for communicating outside of the bedroom or dungeon.

One of the most important lessons we tried to teach men was how to introduce the idea of SM play to their female partner. Having indulged in only isolated masturbatory fantasies of submission, many men may start with some extreme image that has evolved over many years. My advice was not to begin, for instance, with a castration fantasy. That would probably turn her off. Start with something simple and nonthreatening—spanking, perhaps, or gentle scarf bondage. He should ask her about her fantasies instead of focusing only on his own. Many women, for example, have dreamed of a love slave who would service them sexually, but have not put that fantasy into a power context. Introduce the idea of being that love slave by offering a massage or a foot rub, followed by lengthy oral sex if she enjoys that.

Most of all, we say to both parties, stay true to yourself. If the energy is not there, stop. Talk. Try something else. Try again another time. Laugh. Be playful with one another and forgiving of the mis-steps. Remember that it's a mysterious world we enter when we try to actualize erotic fantasy. But it's also a magical sharing of intimate parts of ourselves that can bring us closer together. When it works, it's wonderful.

Tips for Women Wanting to Explore Dominance

* Start with an attitude. Be playful, adventuresome, curious about what you'll learn. Be willing to explore your sexuality, your capacity for sadism. Build your self-confidence with clothing, toys, treats. Love his submission; appreciate your dominance. Maintain your integrity—do it for yourself.

* Trust the energy. Trust the mutuality of the energy—if you're hot, he's hot. Open up the intimate parts of yourself; desire to know his intimate parts as well and don't judge him when he shares them. Look at your dark sides and determine to explore them together—the yin and yang.

* Get yourself turned on first—horny is good! Put yourself in action mode—no lazy dominants. Feel sexy; use your body and hands to tease. Fantasize, fantasize! Find archetypes to emulate: goddess images, powerful women, mothers.

* Create an illusion. Be a "method" actress and find the energy from within. Read his energy and manipulate it. Look into his eyes, watch his cock, check his breathing for clues to his arousal. Plan ahead. Set things up beforehand—surprise him with a new toy, then use it on him.

* Let go of guilt—these energies are natural and positive. See yourself as an object of his desire; know that he wants you! Know that it is a mutually pleasurable expe-

rience. Know that only you can give him what he needs. If you're angry at him, don't play—SM is not real punishment.

* Find the edge, the rush, and follow that energy. Remember him at some level, for safety's sake. Make it real by doing more than he expects, more than you expect. Start where you are comfortable—scratching, light bondage, spanking.

* Create sensation in his body and in yours—pleasure is okay, too. Strip him of control—you take control—forbid a hard-on! Tie his hands behind him. Use body language, facial expressions. Toys are everywhere, in the kitchen, bath, bedroom, fingernails, hair—anything that can create sensation at your command.

* Hypnotize him. Tell him how you want him to be; teach him. Use your voice, making it soft, stern, rhythmically paced. Touch softly; seduce him. Help him relax (very important!). "Spacing out" is profound submission—let him.

* Find out what he likes, what his fantasies are. Have him keep a journal, send you cards with his private thoughts. Decide which of his fantasies you like and use them on him. Give him a ride—the thrill of the roller coaster, a loss of control. Talk to him about what you're going to do to him, and see how he reacts. If there's no charge there, you don't have to follow through.

* Beware of the problems: feeling like his "whore" because you are doing it for him; feeling responsible for his experience and therefore feeling inadequate if it doesn't work; the pressure to be creative (when in doubt, blindfold him); the elusive erection (just because he doesn't get hard doesn't mean he's not excited). Make sure you have "straight" time to be real with each other and talk about the experience.

The Journey to Dark Eros

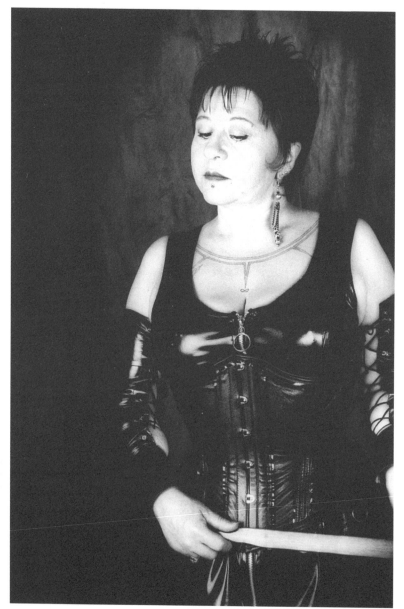

Benjamin Hoffman Photography

Born and raised in Paris, France, Cléo Dubois began exploring the SM frontiers in the San Francisco leather community in the early 1980s. After attending her first, very underground workshop, given by Mistress Kat and Layne, she devoted herself to learning BD (bondage and discipline) and SM skills and safety, as both a top and a bottom. Within a year, she became an enthusiastic, responsible, caring sadist.

Today, with her Academy of SM Arts, Cléo is a highly respected BD/SM educator and Domina, as well as an active member of the San Francisco leather community and a private player. Cléo is a sought-after speaker for such established organizations as Differences, QSM, Society of Janus, NLA Living in Leather conferences, and APEX in Arizona. She is profiled in the book Different Loving.

Carol Queen's in-depth interview of Cléo appeared in the 1998 Bitch Goddess, *edited by Pat Califia and Drew Campbell. She has been featured in magazines* Boudoir Noir, Skin Two, Prometheus, *and the book* Sexual Magic *by Michael A. Rosen. As an educator and body ritual performer she has appeared at London's ICA and at Festival Atlantico in Lisbon, Portugal, and was featured on French television as part of the* Canal+ *series on alternative cultures.*

❋❋❋

Coming out into my sadism and masochism was a powerful and liberating experience for me. I was born and raised in France, where erotic SM has been part of an underground elite culture for centuries. I think, perhaps, that made it easier for me to be proud of my dominant sadism.

As a child, however, I was bullied, dominated, tormented, and humiliated by my male cousins. Power over me was used by my father, my mother, and my peers in an abusive manner. I learned early to distrust and question that sort of authority and to rebel and fight back. As a result I developed inner strength and great independence.

I traveled alone a lot in my early twenties and was outraged at the many ways women were controlled by males in societies governed by patriarchal religions, especially in the Middle East. Whether oppressed by their brothers, fathers, or husbands, women didn't have the right to own their bodies, their sexuality, or even their own pleasure! At that time, I manipulated men through the usual tease and denial tactics learned in my Catholic upbringing.

In 1981, in San Francisco, I attended an SM workshop and immediately found the link to my sexuality that had been missing. My sadism came into focus. Playing with power consensually and erotically made all the difference—this was no longer abuse! In my work today, I help couples and singles with the many skills it takes to safely explore loving bondage and SM role-play. I see this as a way to increase intimacy between players and create what I call "sensual magic" and "the journeys to dark Eros." My expertise and sensitivity enable me to share the secret of successful kinky play; I stress trust, negotiation, turn-on, technical skills, risks and rewards, and the passionate excitement of it all. Since all BD/SM interaction involves negotiation, I first reassure those who contact me that everything they say will remain confidential. A basic lesson I've learned is just how difficult it is for many of us to communicate our erotic needs.

I've learned to ask many questions; the most important one is "What do you mean by that?" I ask what psychological and physical elements are present in the person's fantasy. "Who are you in the fantasy? Are you a willing submissive? A masochist who wants to explore limits? A play slave? A servant? A captive? What sort of activity takes place? Are there any recurring trigger words or images that turn you on?" I do not attempt to act out scripted fantasies, because when people create their fantasies, they are in control of all the elements. When they communicate a fantasy to others, they cannot stay in full control. The acted-out fantasy will never match up to the idea they keep in their heads. I will never be able to take them anywhere real in this kind of situation. Therefore the drama that unfolds must be genuinely collaborative. If I'm only an actress, I don't get a sense of my own power and my intuition is stifled. Having creativity allows me to be powerful and intuitive and keeps the dynamic exciting and hot.

In terms of my own sexuality, playing with an enormous range of people of all ages and from all walks of life has taught me to never say never. It has taught me how rich and diverse are the ways that people express their sexuality. Ten years ago, for example, I had little or no understanding of men who sought to explore their female personae, and even thought that cross-dressing degraded women. Now I appreciate gender role reversal, especially if the situation is kinky and involves a helpless slut or French maid! I've also learned to be aware of the necessity of honoring my own needs as a switch in my private life. Being on the dominant side too much can push me off balance; I know that bottoming in my private life will psychically and erotically recharge me. Unfortunately, I do not have as much desire as I wish I had to top my lovers if they, too, need to be tied up, teased, tormented, and thoroughly done! Another thing that has happened is I've discovered my bisexuality—I cherish the expression of my kinkiness with women as well as with men.

The single most important thing I do to separate the professional SM mistress from my intimate relationship—which I've done from the beginning—is to treat the dungeon as a sacred space, a temple, a sanctuary. What happens in the dungeon happens in a different space, in a different, magical time. It bears no relation to the rest of my life. In addition to this, I maintain certain boundaries with my clients. Like a therapist, I do not socialize with them. I keep my personal and professional lives very separate. I do not work five days a week. I do not, under any circumstances, bottom professionally; I need to keep that space for my private life.

Many people ask how they can get a stranger, or someone new, to open up about their fantasies and live them out in an SM scene. People want to know how to set up boundaries beforehand to make it safe for those involved. If you find yourself in a situation where you are going on a kinky path for the first time with a lover, or perhaps someone you know less well, you need to communicate your fantasies, your expertise, and your experience. What do you want? How compatible are you? How experienced are you? These aren't necessarily easy questions. The SM scene isn't something ready-made that you then act out together. It depends on both parties being able to identify their desires, and to courageously and honestly start expressing them. What do you really want? What does your lover really want? You might not be willing to reveal all the dark, sticky, scary, weird stuff your fantasies are made of. What are you willing to reveal, to explore with this other person? Be clear and brave about what you want and what you are willing to do.

This honesty comes with a risk of rejection: your lover might say no, be horrified or put off. Remember that you have the right to fantasize about whatever you want; fantasy alone never hurt anyone. Being rejected, however, does hurt, so know that it's a possibility. You need to decide who wants to do what to whom. From my long experience with working with couples, I know that it is surprisingly common for lovers to both be switches, or even bottoms. How to negotiate this? Parity, making sure that everyone's needs or desires are met at least some of the time, can mean taking turns. Even though SM people are usually not swingers, but players, they can seek out, with the consent of their partners, other part-time play-partners outside the relationship with whom they can play different games. In most cases, once we've started to really explore our erotic BD/SM desires, it really isn't viable to keep our activities to just one partner.

Now, let's suppose your lover wants to be tied up, but you don't know the first thing about knots. Let's also suppose he or she wants to be spanked for being naughty, and then shamelessly made love to. You might enjoy the idea of making your lover into a slave for the evening, to serve you dessert with a collar around the neck, wearing nothing but a lacy apron and high-heeled shoes.

In the negotiation, find out about any physical limitations your partner may have, such as bad knees or a bad back. Ask about phobias and fears, trigger words that could be hurtful, as well as what they really crave. Give your bottom a safe word. Everyone in California is very familiar with "yellow" for "please slow down, caution, I'm almost at my limit, I need a break," and with "red" for "stop." For the bottom to implore "Please, please stop" is often a turn-on and can be part of the scene, so in determining the safe word it is important to distinguish between fantasy and reality. If you both agree that this could be fun, then this is how to start to play.

Exercise: Your First SM Scene with Someone New

First, set up a special evening for your scene. You'll need a good three or four hours for the whole scene. Instruct your partner on what to wear and what to bring with them. Ask them to find and buy a frilly apron and some sexy high-heeled shoes. Have your equipment ready too.

For this scene, you'll need a dog collar that fits your bottom's neck and an attachable chain—which can be found

at the supermarket or in a leather store—and perhaps
some light bondage wrist-cuffs and a sleep-mask or a
blindfold. Also obtain a piece of nylon rope no longer than
three yards, and not too thin—twine can cut. Look around
the kitchen and see what else catches your eye. A wooden
kitchen spoon makes a great spanking implement, as does
a small wooden cutting board or a wooden back-scratcher
if you have one. Find some clothespins to use as nipple
clamps. Have fun thinking of erotic uses for everyday
household objects!

Unplug the phone. Set the scene with some low lighting,
maybe some candles, and some sensuous or evocative
music. If you want a more Victorian feel, play some
Mozart. Pick your costume carefully (you might, at some
point, order your slave to undress you and to fold your
clothes neatly, while remaining on her or his hands and
knees).

Find a comfortable seat, take a few deep breaths, be centered, and call in your slave. Tell him or her to come close
to you and be seen. Have him or her slowly undress before
you and fold their clothes in a neat pile on the floor. Have
him or her drop to hands and knees and put the clothes to
one side while you watch him or her crawl. Comment on
his or her form and beauty, like you would a fine new
acquisition. Caress your new toy gently and slowly.

Order him or her to kneel before you. Take the collar in
your hands. Stand up and ask if he or she is ready to
accept your collar as a symbol of willing submission. Say
how you wish to be addressed: Sir, Madam, My Lady,
Lord, Master, or Mistress. Ask him or her to tell you what
the safe words are, to ensure everyone remembers. Take
control of your slave's actions. Do you want his or her
eyes lowered to the floor or looking up at you? Keep your
orders simple and precise. See how they are followed. Be
just: if your slave is good and attentive, he or she should
be rewarded, touched sweetly, turned on.

If the service is bad, if your drink is spilled, give your slave five good whacks with the wooden spoon. It is possible that your partner might be sassy and even seek some light humiliation or more pain. How does that feel? Don't get angry; remember that you are both playing. It's only by experimenting with acting out your fantasy that you will discover who your play persona is—master, trainer, inter-rogator, brat, good girl/boy, smart-ass masochist, or true submissive slave.

Play and have fun. You might want to place the clothes-pins on your slave's nipples just to see how he or she responds to a little pain. Make sure you look into your partner's eyes when you remove them after a few minutes, and take notice of your own reaction—could you have a sadistic streak? You might want to use the rope to tie your submissive's hands behind his or her back or to a chair, or cuff and tie him or her to the bed. Simple knots are always the best, and make sure to have a pair of scissors handy just in case.

Blindfolding your bound lover and tormenting him or her with gentle sensual touching will heighten the perception of your touch. Playing with trust and surrender in this way can be a fabulous turn-on. Your hands, your voice, your mouth, your breath are also your toys, so use them to full effect. Your power doesn't come from the rope or wooden spoon, but from you. All these things are but extensions of your power and energy, emanating from your core. Be cen-tered, feel your power, feel the turn-on that you create for yourself and your partner.

Be open to the exchange of energy between the two of you. Try shifting the power around; get really close to your bot-tom, whisper softly, touch sweetly, breathe warm breath on your lover's neck. Stand apart, take charge with your voice, run your nails across his or her skin. Use contrasts in sen-sations. Your hands can touch sweetly, but can also rub, pinch, and scratch. Don't ask for permission. Pay atten-tion to the responses, your partner's breathing and level of turn-on.

Don't be shy to ask specifically for what you really want your bottom to do for you. Maybe you want your breasts touched and kissed in a certain way. Perhaps you wish your lover to worship your feet and ankles. Tell him or her exactly how you like it, how you want it done. Guide your partner so he or she can serve you in the best possible way. Be present for the turn-on that brings. Use breathing techniques to keep centered: deep breathing increases awareness of our being in our bodies and makes it easier to project our power outward. In this way you create a ritualized, magical scene. I strongly believe in the magic of SM and intimacy games.

Find your power. Feel it, use it, play with it, and above all, enjoy it. This scene might not have much heavy SM or bondage, and maybe it will lead to some great, hot straight sex, but that's just the point. You've opened the door, gotten a taste, and the future is wide open. Remember, you collared your partner as a symbol of your dominance and his or her submission. It is your responsibility to remove it and to close the scene when the play is ended. Talking about the scene the next day, or within a few days, is also very important.

Exploring our fantasy lives can raise questions of what is consensual power play and what is real abuse. The SM credo, as is well-known, is that play must be safe, sane, and consensual. Nonetheless, many things can happen in the context of a scene when limits are reached and challenged. Emotional damage often cannot be anticipated. A certain judgment made in a scene might cut like a knife to the heart; our fears over our inadequacies might be powerfully and painfully triggered; our high can turn into a painful dive into depression and fear of rejection. This can be equally true from a top or a bottom perspective.

In terms of physical damage, what's important is to be educated about what is and isn't safe to play with. There is a great deal of concrete information out there, both in nonfiction books and on the World Wide Web.

Nothing to Fear

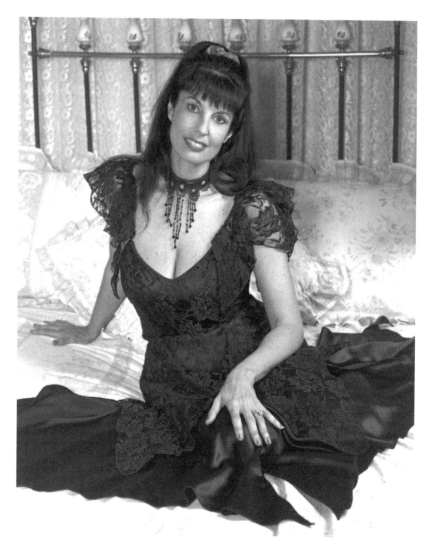

Amanda Dwyer began her career as a mistress in 1986 with an apprenticeship at Salon Kitty's in Sydney, which had been established four months earlier as a brothel. It soon began specializing in BD and fantasy services, with a core of experienced mistresses from around Sydney.

Amanda's natural flair and attraction to SM, plus her sense of organization and former business experience, soon resulted in her coming to the notice of Salon Kitty's owner. What was intended to be a dalliance with the scene turned into a management position within the establishment. In 1989, she bought the business outright.

Like most people who are into the SM scene, dominance and submission had been part of Amanda's psyche from an early age. Like many people, she was unable to recognize this until she saw an advertisement for apprentice mistresses. She responded to the ad, and spending one day among the extraordinary women who are mistresses and submissives in a professional establishment was enough to convince her.

Amanda has advocated for the BD and SM scene and the sex industry in general. In 1990, Amanda was part of a movement aimed at legalizing and legitimizing the sex industry in New South Wales and for a year was the industry's main spokesperson.

Amanda has often been called the Queen of BDSM in Australia, but she still continues to conduct sessions at Salon Kitty's. After thirteen years in the profession, one-to-one sessions remain the most important expression of her SM life. She says, "It has become my business, but most importantly, it is a fundamental part of my personality."

✳✳✳

I have appeared repeatedly in the media in an educational role, not to evangelize BD and SM, but to demystify it. I believe it is a form of expression important to only a minority of people, but to those people it is a crucial part of life. I have always sought to demonstrate that there is nothing to fear from BD or SM. As long as the basic tenets of "safe, sane, and consensual" are followed, then BD and SM are just expressions of human sexuality and interaction.

I don't think my work has been good for my own sexuality. I think I have become so centered on being obliged to constantly give pleasure to others that in my own private life I tend to get a bit over it all. My life revolves around hearing and reading, supplying and satisfying men's sexual fantasies. I think it is easy to become a little jaded. I think a lot of what I have experienced over the years makes me realize there are and always will be many differences between men and women on matters of sexual feelings and interest. I know I haven't found all the answers to what gives me a sexual high.

At this point in my life I feel as though I have totally lost touch with my sexuality. I know a lot of women say they don't really know or understand themselves sexually until they reach the age of thirty-five, but I can't say the same goes for me. It isn't that I haven't grown or learned anything over the years, but I do blame my work for interfering with my personal sexual expression. I think by constantly having to satisfy in a commercial sense (no matter what role you may be taking), you take on the mindset of having to deliver, and you feel there is always something expected from you.

These expectations (which I put upon myself) tend to invade my personal life. I think I have become afraid of finding my real sexual self. I wouldn't say working in the sex industry has done a great deal for my personal confidence. I think you need to have a certain amount of confidence to feel, and actually be, sexy. Contrary to popular belief, not all who work in the BD/SM scene have the confidence many people assume we possess.

I don't believe women are the superior sex or that any woman is a goddess. I do believe women should have rights and opportunities equal to men's. We are an equal part of the human race, yet we still strive to be recognized in many societies today. Some attitudes will take several generations to change.

Tips for Safely Exploring BD/SM Within Your Relationship

* First of all, it is necessary that both parties are interested and want to be involved. The words "safe, sane, and consensual" are paramount. You must be able to trust your partner; without trust this style of relationship should not be entered into.

* Most people like to take either the dominant or submissive role. I believe it is a good idea when first starting out to try taking on both roles in turns. Most of us have a natural tendency to be dominant or submissive, but it never hurts to know just how it feels both physically and emotionally to be in either position.

* It is always important to start off by taking things

slowly. It is also a good idea not to try too many activities in the first session, as it could be a little overwhelming. BD/SM is a very sexual experience, but it produces arousal of a type that you have probably never experienced before.

* Try sensory deprivation. It is amazing how the body feels when you are lightly restrained and unable to hear or see. Physical sensations seem to increase dramatically.

* Many people find it difficult to actually put their feelings or desires into words for fear of rejection or disapproval. It is paramount that people inform partners of their levels of interest and experience, and that they obey and respect each other's limits.

* Purchase a few basic items from your local sex shop. Wrist and/or ankle restraints, a slave collar that signifies the submissive position, a blindfold for sensory deprivation (this can heighten sexual awareness), some sash cord for basic bondage, long shoelaces for genital bondage, a small leather paddle, and a riding crop. Clothespins can be substituted for nipple clamps (which can be quite expensive). These items are very basic but won't break the budget.

* If you find you like exploring these roles, you can purchase other pieces of equipment and discipline implements. Some creative individuals get a lot of fun from making their own toys and equipment. If you fall into this category all the better; handmade pieces are far more personal.

* Finally, once you feel confident in your chosen role, you may like to venture a little further by attending BD or SM functions where you can meet like-minded people who share your interests. These gatherings can be lots of fun and a good way to make new friends.

PART 7

Oral Sex and Female Ejaculation

Traditionally, sex workers have been viewed as victims—women who have endured tragic childhoods, are generally unloved, or are victims of an unscrupulous man or a serious drug habit. There has been little acceptance of the possibility that a woman could choose sex work as a short-term or long-term career option and make a success of it. More shocking is the view that women could enjoy sex work or be prostitutes or dominatrices as well as loving wives and caring mothers.

Many women who have never worked in the sex industry are fascinated by the world's oldest profession. For women to watch a strip show or a live erotic performance is to see another woman wield her sexual power in a way that can be erotic and seductive. For many women the sexual fantasy of being a prostitute, from a high-class whore to a sassy streetwalker, is a way of playing with being wanted and desired. When a woman fantasizes about being a leather-clad dominatrix with her own dungeon of gorgeous slaves, she can experience absolute power and control.

To be both a feminist and a sex worker is even more controversial, to feminists and nonfeminists alike. It is the feminist sex workers who have offered some of the most important new insights into the sex industry. Unfortunately, they have also been the women most attacked by other women as betraying the feminist cause, because they see no contradiction between wanting to overthrow male power and running a sexual service for men.

Many sex workers have to live with the stigma still attached to sex work, meaning they often are forced to lead a double life. The stress of having to cover up what you do for a living, and the fear of being found out, can cause extreme personal pressure for individual sex workers. It is important that movements for sexual liberation include rights for sex workers to empowerment and legalization or decriminalization of the industry.

For some women, working in the sex industry has been a negative experience they regret; for others, their time in the industry has been a way to learn about human sexuality. Sex workers get a unique look at people's fantasies, insecurities, vulnerabilities, and fears. They are frontline sexual researchers and have an untapped body of knowledge that should be respected and documented. Most of them would not give up their sex-industry experiences—either good or bad—for the world.

In this part, two women who know—both of them professionals in the sex industry—reveal their very different perspectives. They also share the expertise they've spent years accumulating. They offer techniques: one for pleasing the woman in your life, and the other for thrilling your man.

Female ejaculation does exist! My first hand experience occurred in a workshop for sexual exploration and was beautifully demonstrated by a lesbian couple. One woman graciously demonstrated her amazing technique by placing a finger inside her partner's vagina and moving it against the G-spot. I was delighted when I saw the urethral sponge come down from the vagina, becoming visible as clear liquid ejaculated.

The G-spot was first named by Ernest Graffenberg in the 1940s and has been a controversial subject for many years. Some people believe it to be the female equivalent of the male prostate. It is a cluster of nerve endings and glands which is part of the urethral sponge. When it is stimulated, it can produce a secretion of clear liquid that is often mistaken for urine. This process is known as female ejaculation.

To find the G-spot, place a finger into the vagina and push it forward towards the stomach. Approximately 2" in you will feel skin with a ribbed or rougher texture than the surrounding tissue. This is the G-Spot and it can be anywhere from a half inch to an inch and a half in size. As a woman becomes sexually aroused, the tissue swells with blood and makes this area more sensitive. The G-spot can also be a place where sexual trauma can be lodged.

Not all women will experience ejaculation; it will depend on the style of orgasm she has. A clitoral orgasm has an emphasis on warm energy going up the body, while female ejaculation is a release of energy with women experiencing a pushing down sensation. To help to learn to ejaculate, use a variation of exercising your genital muscles by clenching, relaxing, and gently pushing out your genital muscles, then relax and push out again. Repeat this as often as possible, approximately two hundred times a day.

Sexuality pioneer Deborah Sundahl demystified the G-spot orgasm and female ejaculation through her best-selling video, *How to Female Ejaculate*. Her clear explanations and cheeky how-to sessions offered a new, lucid insight into this previously little-understood phenomenon. Sexually fulfilling a woman by stimulating her G-spot is something every lover of women should know and every woman should experience. Sundahl's video and her work in this area are the kind of public sexuality education we need. Here, Deborah Sundahl shares her extraordinary journey from publisher of erotica to spiritual sensualist.

Every sex worker knows about oral sex, a standard stock-in-trade for the professional. It is the number one fantasy of most men, and the ability of sex workers to fulfill this dream is highly prized. Dolores French, who still works in the sex industry, gives a professional's humorous perspective on blow jobs and offers expert tips.

Spiritual Access

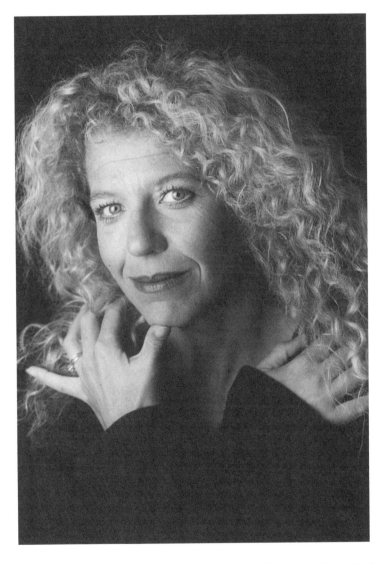

American-born Deborah Sundahl was one of the founders of On Our Backs, *a lesbian erotic magazine that ran for ten years, from 1984 to 1994. It was the mouthpiece for emerging women's erotica—women speaking their sexual desires*

in their own voice. Many women credit the magazine for changing their lives, and it was the inspiration for many other women's erotic magazines.

She was also well-known as San Francisco stripper extraordinaire Fanny Fatale, with her own loyal following. She pioneered the women-only strip shows Burlezk *and brought the art of striptease to a female-only audience.*

She is currently producer of women's educational sex videos, which she describes as "erotica with intelligence and spirit from a woman's point of view." She specializes in educating about Tantric sex and female ejaculation.

✳✳✳

On Our Backs was the first magazine to address sexuality positively and from a woman's point of view. All other magazines at that time were created by men for men's enjoyment. *On Our Backs* addressed important sexual issues for women, such as broadening the definition of the female body, enjoying sex toys, allowing and expressing one's fantasies, exploring gender-bending (role reversals), and dominant-submissive play.

The point with *On Our Backs* was to have fun with sex, educate ourselves about the variety of sexual expressions possible in order to foster tolerance, and shed the personal guilt that kept us from our true sexual desires. As a lesbian magazine, *On Our Backs* flew in the face of the conservative, antisex lesbian culture that existed at the time, and which mimicked the larger culture's conservative swing. The magazine was liberating and lively and broke sexual taboos continuously in its initial years.

By the time I sold the magazine in 1994, *On Our Backs* had created real cultural change. Sexuality was recognized as the defining force that broadened and unified a newly emerging culture, which included not just lesbians, but gay men, bisexuals, and hip heterosexual couples. The ideas in *On Our Backs* also began to seep into a stagnant, male-dominated adult sex industry. Women, both gay and straight, were beginning to have influence for the first time as consumers over what was made and purchased, and they demanded quality.

It was out of this context of destroying old, damaging stereotypes of female sexuality and birthing new definitions of ourselves from our truth that I suddenly hit a huge wall in my own sexuality. After I left *On Our Backs* my libido bit the dust, which meant I had nothing more to say or to create with. I had been on the forefront of female sexuality, and now I began to question all I had taught and publicized for ten years. I felt like I was disintegrating, my identity being stripped from me. It was incredibly terrifying, and I felt as raw as someone without skin. I sought out the solace and protection of the deserts of the southwestern United States to go through this change and sort things out.

The Southwest is a very spiritual place—rich in Native American culture—and not very populated. There, I could reflect in solitude and anonymity. It became clear that what had started out as a labor of love and intense creativity had turned into a soul-draining management headache. I was juggling publication deadlines, the horrendous cash flow endemic to small counterculture projects, and the video production and mail-order parts of the business. We tried to grow the business, using every tenacious skill we had, but we failed. It was a difficult time, and I sold the magazine. I had given all I had, and enough was enough. Sitting under a star-filled night, a refugee from the city culture, I began the slow process of diving deep and surfacing with real parts of my lost self.

What began to emerge was a passion for nature and learning to be responsible for my own survival. I began a research trip, visiting and working on permaculture and herb farms and assisting with the building of alternative structures. I learned I had far greater capability to care for myself than our medical establishment and economic structure would like us to believe. When I first stepped into a house made completely of organic materials from the earth, heated and powered by the sun, watered by the rains, and cleaned by the plants, the nurturing feeling was so overwhelming that I sat down and sobbed.

Meanwhile, my libido had degenerated to the point where I could not touch myself sexually without feeling terribly devastated or lethargic. I knew something new was emerging, requiring me to reject all my well-worn, playful and joyful, nasty and lusty ways. I followed an impulse to practice yoga daily, and this led to an exploration of "devotional love." In devotional yoga, one meditates on the subtle feelings, both emotional and physical, that arise in the body while in a yoga position.

One day, to my great surprise, my libido leaped into a raging fire as I sat immersed in contemplation of uniting myself with the cosmic force. So I meditated on these sexual feelings, as I did with all the other feelings that arose in my body. I experimented with "hold-ing" as much erotic pleasure as possible, and with foregoing the urge, almost instinctive in most of us, to immediately satisfy it. There was a period when I moved to Santa Fe, New Mexico, when I did this for hours at a time. I found a place on the edge of a forest where I could meditate in silence, and I lived like a hermit for two years. The forest, ancient growth in particular, is where my power as a woman lies, and it is fuelled by my sexuality. My spirit is powered and directed by my erotic energy.

Getting in touch with my sexual desires and emotions and giv-ing them voice for all those years has obviously led me to desiring to feel the voice of the earth and the whispers of the forest. To express my sexuality and love for another in that context is awesome and exciting and feels like a vast frontier. I have had to be unpart-nered all this time to peel away the old sexuality and birth the new self. I look forward to sharing this greater capacity to express my sexuality in a spiritual context with a new partner someday soon.

After many years of painstaking inner searching, I was able to leave my hermitage. I found I had gained new purpose and renewed strength and recharged vitality to take with me back out into the work world. The message I gained was clear: uncovering our sexual fantasies, becoming "erotically literate" about ourselves, and gaining the confidence to successfully communicate our sexual needs all lead to uncovering the real power of our erotic being: spiritual access. This is self-knowledge of a very deep kind. At its core, sexual expression is about learning how to love ourselves and others.

I used to laugh at this concept of love in the early stages of *On Our Backs*, thinking it too gooey and stereotypical of what a woman was expected to be. At *On Our Backs* we felt it was essential that women loosen up sexually and behave more aggressively. For instance, bend that guy over and drop his pants and do a quickie with a dildo and harness. This sojourn into an all-stops-pulled sex-ual exploration led me, full circle, back to love. It required a more sobering look at what that feels like in my body, and what that kind of intimacy with another actually requires.

Recently, Gina Odgen, a colleague and author of the book *Women Who Love Sex*, pointed out that perhaps I had been doing this more intimate, spiritually based loving all along, but simply had not the words to describe or define it as such. I realized that the tenderness and intimacy I felt when embraced in an SM scene was profound. Can one really understand surrender if one has never had one's hands and feet bound and lain helpless in complete trust of the one they love? I have used those experiences to practice surrendering into the tenderness and bliss of someone loving me or of myself loving me.

Back in the work world, I considered doing a heterosexual couples' version of my best-selling video *How to Female Ejaculate*, knowing it would sell well and get me back on my feet, but my artistic self refused. Instead, the video *Journey to Female Orgasm: Awakening the G-spot and Female Ejaculation* was born. I felt it necessary to record this incredible process of transformation and to help women take those first few steps toward accessing the world of spiritual-sexual power. The video demonstrates how the G-spot is not a magic button for instant gratification, but is instead the opposite: a source of intense physical sensation and deep emotions, and a gateway to accessing consciousness.

This is important news about the G-spot, and in the video *Journey to Female Orgasm* I explain how a G-spot massage can heal these old traumatic wounds to our sexual seat and reawaken it to its true and powerful potential. When I made *How to Female Ejaculate* in 1991, I feared I'd be run out of town on a rail for saying that all woman can ejaculate, because the phenomenon was so utterly silenced that few people knew about it. Those women who did ejaculate usually mistook it for peeing in bed and suffered awful embarrassment and shame. Sometimes their husbands left them, or they simply stopped without being aware that they had the capability to control ejaculation.

Ejaculation, in women and men, can be controlled. Women have learned to control it almost completely and men have learned to control it hardly at all. This is a huge sexual imbalance between the sexes that Tantric practices have done much to correct.

Today, female ejaculation is more understood and even popularized, so I want to take it to the next level. This level parallels my sexual process from political liberation to spiritual awakening. A new century is upon us that demands we live on this earth and treat ourselves and others on a much higher, loving level than we have so far. Sexuality is a path to learning this. It makes perfect sense to me that sexuality and its inherent power have been silenced, suppressed, cajoled, and repulsed, for sexuality is the root of our life force. A mindset that creates a culture of death and violence cannot allow a vital life force to direct individuals. Instead of buying into that mindset, awaken the hidden potential of your G-spot and female ejaculation with the following exercise.

Exercise: Accessing the Erotic Spiritual Realm

No alcohol, marijuana, or drugs of any kind are to be used for at least seventy-two hours before the exercise. This entire erotic meditation can be done with or without a partner. In either case, allow three hours for the exercise.

Find a wilderness setting in warm, sunny weather near a creek on a warm, moonlit evening, with or without a fire. A private, quiet, outdoor setting is essential for this exercise, as you are about to access higher consciousness. Bring a cock ring or cock-and-ball strap for him and Ben-Wa balls or preferably a finished gemstone, golf-ball-sized, for her. Bring a thick, padded blanket and two pillows, a charcoal burner, and sage and frankincense. Bring an icon of your choice, perhaps Isis, Lilith, Shiva, Pan, or the Horned God. Bring a journal or sketch pad, chocolate, and water. Bring matches.

Remove your clothes. Light the incense and sage. Smudge the smoke of the lit sage over your bodies to lighten up your energy and purify it of negative thoughts and emotions. Look into each other's eyes as you cleanse and prepare each other with the sage. Put on the cock ring and insert the stone ball into the vagina. Then say the following centering prayer, or one of your choice: "Let this sacred act be protected by the gods. Let this sacred act of love fly in the wind in gratitude to that which gives us life. Let this sacred act in which we are about to partake nourish us and all energy around us."

Sit face to face, hold hands, and cross your legs around

149

Oral Sex
and
Female
Ejacula-
tion

each other in a comfortable position. Meditate on the feelings that arise in your body. Repeat the following ten times, very slowly, like a mantra: "Pleasure is love and I am opening to pleasure. Pleasure is love and I am opening to pleasure. Pleasure is love and I am opening to pleasure." Allow your body to express its physical sensations, and stay "present," that is, fully aware of them. Meditate on the sensations that well up, such as in your chest or stomach or loins. Move if a part of your body wants to move. Let it lead as you keep the mind focused on the mantra and on the body's voice of feeling and movement talking to you. The practice is about having complete trust in the process and in the guidance you are receiving through your body.

The female partner can touch her male partner's perineum, which is situated between his anus and testicles. At the same time, he can gently hold her nipples with his fingertips or take this time to relax and meditate on giving and receiving love. Repeat, "This is what love feels like. This is what love feels like. This is what love feels like." Start to move your fingers very slowly and concentrate on making your touch emulate your love feelings and allowing this to expand. Whenever the love feeling goes away and gets replaced with the urge to satisfy the erotic sensations, stop all stimulation and contact.

Recenter and refocus on the love feeling and start again. Each time, you will expand the area of your lover's body you are touching as you refocus on the feeling of love. After six times or so of stopping and starting, depending on your experience and ability to hold focus and pleasure and love, you have made it to the point where the man can massage his female partner's G-spot.

Here is the point at which the G-spot can be truly awakened to its full potential, as the gateway to intense physical sensations of love, deep-seated emotions, and mystical states of consciousness. The woman may wish to receive the massage, although it is possible for both partners to give and receive at the same time. Be aware to stop when-ever the pleasure cascades over into sensations of lust and relax the breath by breathing deeply, then begin again, recentered on the love feeling.

Let sensations and emotions surface, and acknowledge them by saying: "I welcome you. You are the truth in me. Be voiced." If at any time emotions have to be expressed or the intimacy becomes too intense and uncomfortable, sim-ply stop. Express the emotions with your partner. This is done in turns as one person speaks and the other listens. You may wish to recite an erotic, devotional love prayer: "I receive from you pure love and return its healing energy with joy." Each person can repeat this three times. Lie (or sit) entwined and keep turning the feelings of pleasure into love.

Remember to discontinue all movement if the sensations of love get lost to the sexual urge. Eye contact is essential. You will at some point enter orgasmic bliss, completely enveloped in this feeling of love, or the erotic love feelings will dissipate into a feeling of full satisfaction as if you had orgasmed. Either way will be utterly divine.

You may find through this process that you feel an altered state of consciousness, made obvious by a heightened sense of hearing, sight, or other sensory awareness. Com-mune with nature, experiment with breathing with the trees, or listen to the rocks or wind. This is where the practice ends and where your personal experience and path begin. You are on your own, finding your own truth, using your union with your partner to become one with the other beings around you.

After thirty to ninety minutes, you will regain your usual sense of reality. End the session with a sage smudge and a prayer of gratitude to the cosmos and to each other. Eat the chocolate and drink the water. Write down or sketch your impressions of the experience. Snuggle up and nap or go to sleep for the evening.

A Little Way Out, a Little Way In

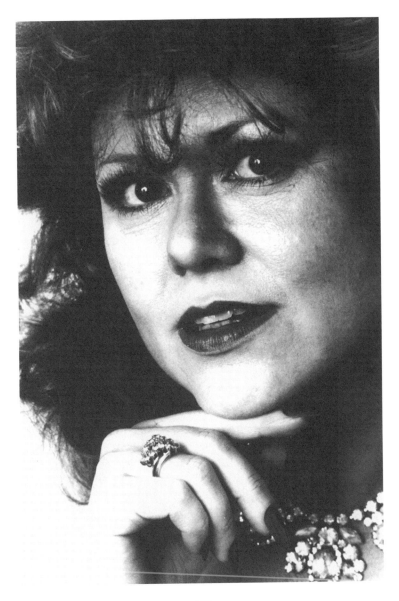

Dolores French was born in 1951 in Kentucky. She studied journalism and photography and eventually moved into radio, working in management at a radio station.

She has worked as a prostitute all around the world. After all the traveling she has done, she loves being at home in Georgia, where her work consists of phone sex, specializing in domination. She also writes for Hustler *magazine.*

Dolores is presently working on a couple of books, writes columns for the magazines Vixen *and* The Scene, *and is a regular television and radio commentator on the sex industry.*

❋❋❋

I still work as a prostitute and have regular clients who I have been seeing for twenty years. If I go for a week without seeing anyone, it's not good, as I really enjoy my work. I never want to retire. I see the way I work now as different from when I first started, because I am more comfortable with myself.

I feel very comfortable with my body, and I find that men are grateful to be with someone who is sexual and skilled. Men are not as critical of women's bodies as women are. Sexually, I am so much better now than when I was in my twenties. I remember when I was that age working with a woman who was in her late forties or early fifties, and I knew I would never be as sexy as she was until I reached her age. She had a sensuality and an artistic approach to sexuality, and she was so graceful in her approach. I have a sexiness now that I could not have had earlier in my life.

I have many relationships in my life, both sexual and nonsexual. Many people find my relationship with my husband odd, but I would not have involved myself with him to begin with if he were not open to the person I am. I would advise partners who want to introduce other people into their relationship to be open and honest and to really understand the boundaries and commitments of your relationship.

Being very clear does not mean cornering your partner into an agreement about how to operate the relationship that is not really in his or her heart. If I were to make an agreement with my husband to have a monogamous relationship it would never work, because that is not in my heart. Being up-front and honest about that is so important. Sex is such a small part of the whole relationship, and expecting it to be the thing that either holds a relationship together or dissolves it is stupid, I think.

153

Oral Sex
and
Female
Ejacula-
tion

When addressing the issue of monogamy at the International Conference on Prostitution, zoologist Robin Baker told us that human sperm is specialized. Perhaps fourteen different types of sperm each do a very specialized task, one of which is to kill. Baker proposed that these sperm have been genetically programmed to assassinate others because they "expect" to find other sperm from other males in any given vagina or uterus.

Baker also pondered an interesting observation about the shape of the penis. Why is that tip there, anyway? Apparently, Baker says, it is to act as a plunger, to suck out the other guy's semen during the back-and-forth, in-and-out motion.

My Face Has Fallen and It Can't Get Up

Recently, I have been considering plastic surgery, and after a visit to a specialist I had an insight into the physically beneficial effects of my years performing professional oral sex.

I explained to the doctor, Rod Hester, that I just wanted my chin and eyes tucked. Then he started showing me how they could restore my whole face. It was impressive. He did it all with his fingers, not on one of those computer-imaging things. I think the computer-imaging things are fun, but I'm suspicious of the results—after all, Fred Astaire dances with a Broom Vac™ via computer imaging. Besides, I've got plenty of images of where different parts of my face used to be—they're called photographs. Anyway, with just his fingers the doctor was able to put all the pieces back to where they once were.

It gave me nostalgic longings, sentimental memories of tight elasticity. Gone are the days when fellatio held my flesh tightly in place on my face. As Rod poked at my jaws and jowls and speculated about restoring cheekbone definition, I wondered if maybe doing a six-week stint sucking cocks in the Caribbean couldn't do the same thing. This is something I can't stop thinking about: the physical benefits of cheap whorehouse life. I was in great condition when I worked those places.

In the 1980s I wrote the following about fellatio: "If I didn't do it every day my tongue got tired, my jaws got tired, my lips got tired. When I went home for a little rest and recreation in Atlanta, however, everyone commented about how the structure of my face seemed to have changed. My cheeks seemed leaner, my jawline tighter. I knew it was from giving head." Back here in the slash-and-suck world of cosmetic surgery, Rod was doing a good job of showing me how he could cut here and tuck there and suck a little out here and inject it there and in about six hours make my face as good as new, almost. A mini brow-lift would be the crowning touch.

I could see that he was right, though I never lost sight of the benefits blow jobs could offer. Still, I could see that while the fellatio treatment could cure a lot of ailments, surgery was the only solution to some of the problems.

Now it was time to see the appointment secretary, Libby, about scheduling all this and paying for it. She was a cute young woman with a cute, even-younger nose. After all her figuring, including the overnight stay in the recovery suite, Libby announced the total cost would be (are you ready for your own mini brow-lift?) $14,025! Libby immediately added that, in my case, the mini brow-lift might not be absolutely necessary, bringing the cost down to about $12,000.

My daily affirmation became, "I have a spare $15,000 for cosmetic surgery. I have a spare $15,000 for cosmetic surgery. I have a spare $15,000 for cosmetic surgery."

Health insurance doesn't cover such procedures, I'm told. Who decides these things? While I'm doing no more than walking around upright on this planet, I'm being victimized by gravity! If falling flesh doesn't count as an accident, who decides what does? Maybe the same nitwits who lobby legislation defining the difference between bestiality and professional animal breeding. What brilliant philosopher proposed that it's legal to jerk off dogs, horses, etc., as long as it's for profit, but it's illegal and immoral if it's just good fun for all involved? I want a head count of the elected idiots that voted this professional dog pimping into law. There's no doubt in my mind that it's the same bunch of befuddled people who came up with these health insurance policies.

If you can spare $15,000 for my beautification/historical-restoration project, e-mail me at Frenchdom@aol.com. Donations are not tax deductible. And to learn the fellatio method for nipping and tucking—which will buy you a little time, at least—read on.

Exercise: The Best Blow Job

I perfected the best way to do a blow job in the Caribbean. The women I worked with would sit around waiting for the next client and discussing the best methods to suck a guy off in the least possible time. Some believed you should suck hard, or that tongue flicks were the answer; others thought deep throating or using an up-and-down speed was it. Another woman believed that placing a finger in the anus made it the best, while another was adamant it was all the moaning-and-slurping sound effects that did it. I tried each of these methods and realized that none by itself was the answer. But when I put them all together and found my own natural rhythm, men found it amazingly exciting.

I learned a lot from the way Japanese men make love. They don't just go in and out; they make a pattern of it. They go in, a little way out, a little way in, a little way out, a little out, a little out, way in, in, in. I adopted this rhythm into the way I gave blow jobs. I teased, stroked, and added a sudden surprise of tickling as the man relaxed into deep pleasure. I got rave reviews from clients and a lot of repeat business. And usually it took no longer than seven minutes for my clients to come.

PART 8

Film and Pornography

Hollywood movies of the last decade showed more sex than ever before; explicit lovemaking scenes, masturbation, and even homo-erotic encounters are no longer uncommon. Television portrayals of sexuality are also increasingly explicit, with the high-rated soap operas showing (or at least implying) not just sexy encounters between married couples, but also casual affairs, sex between strangers, and even the odd ménage à trois. We've come a long way from *Leave It to Beaver.*

People see so much sex in mainstream media now that it is not surprising they want even more explicit imagery. X-rated videos are readily available to fulfill this wish. The video porn industry is rela-tively new, only as old as the video recorder itself, so people's ability to buy or rent porn movies for private use is a new phenomenon. The home video recorder also has allowed people to star in their own erotic escapades. The X-rated video industry has burgeoned, and in the United States the Kinsey Institute has estimated that one in three videos rented is X-rated.

In a typical X-rated video the focus is on genital action rather than on the story line or the emotional interplay between characters. Women have long been critical of the X-rated video industry, to the point of campaigning to have such videos banned or claiming that they contribute to violence against women, including rape. Other women have not accepted the charge that explicit porn causes vio-lence, but have criticized the fact that women's sexual pleasure is frequently ignored and that women are often portrayed in demean-ing ways. In fairness, while pornography can be said to reflect the views of society, including its stereotypical views of women, it can-not be blamed for creating them.

156

Free-speech activists, some of whom are also feminists, have argued that censorship is not the answer. Rather, women taking some degree of control within the industry is a better solution. They claim that an eager market exists for sexually explicit adult films geared toward women and couples, markets that have been traditionally ignored. They argue that films can be sexually hot yet still reflect a progressive view of women who are in charge of their sexuality and their lives.

By the mid-1980s this theory was put into practice. Independent erotic-video makers started producing porn for women and couples, as well as lesbian-made porn for lesbians. And it sold. Former porn star Candida Royalle swapped places for a role on the other side of the lens and produced a best-selling string of movies for women and couples. The publishers of the lesbian sex magazine *On Our Backs* launched a video line, Fatale Films. These video companies continue to exist and have gone from strength to strength. Other independent female video companies also produced new-style erotica, and the old-boys' porn network eventually caught on and started producing videos for the couples market.

The popularity of the new porn produced by companies run by women has shown that this is the direction of the future. The videos contain nudity and graphic depictions of sex, but no coercion or violence. They also place emphasis on a woman's sexual pleasure and give a realistic depiction of women's sexuality. Although these new porn pioneers have less capital than the mainstream producers, they spend up to ten times more on their films.

Women are also at the forefront of another type of erotic video: sex-education videos that show and describe what makes sex better, without deliberate erotic titillation. When women started exploring the G-spot and female ejaculation, it became obvious that there was only so far one could go without explicit visual demonstration. The same video-porn pioneers produced the new sex-education videos, which proved to have the same eager audience. Videos on female ejaculation, Tantric sex, anal pleasure for men, and safe sex for women and couples were eagerly sought for their no-nonsense, sex-positive approach—and their sense of humor.

Women who work within the porn industry are now less closeted about their professions than previously, with stars such as Nina Hartley crossing over to Hollywood in the film *Boogie Nights*. They have set up support systems for each other and created a sisterhood within the sex industry. The development of women's visual imagery, including video, has been an essential component of women's sexual empowerment. It provides a way of duplicating what women see in the best relationships, from how to seduce someone to how to touch and caress a lover.

Statistics of porn-video rentals show that people frequently seek erotic material that is outside their sexual preference. Straight women rent movies of gay men, lesbians rent films depicting bisexual ménages à trois, and straight men (famously) rent lesbian videos. Every survey shows that while some people regard society as becoming more conservative, a large percentage of the general public wants the right to have sexually explicit material available to consenting adults in their own homes. Video sales show that the popularity of porn is not waning.

Despite the political and legal battles that continue around classification and censorship, personal issues remain for couples who wish to enjoy X-rated videos together. Many people feel embarrassed to bring up their desire to watch a porn video with their partner; some fear that letting their partner know what they fantasize about exposes their sexual vulnerability. Others worry that the exoticism of the onscreen scenario compares unfavorably with their own domesticity. Beautiful porn stars and those with impossible endowments can cause partners to feel uneasy about their own bodies.

In this part, Nan Kinney addresses these issues and describes how to have a romantic porn-video date, and Candida Royalle and Nina Hartley reveal what life is really like in the porn industry.

Fantasies: A Reflection of What Is Happening in Our Life

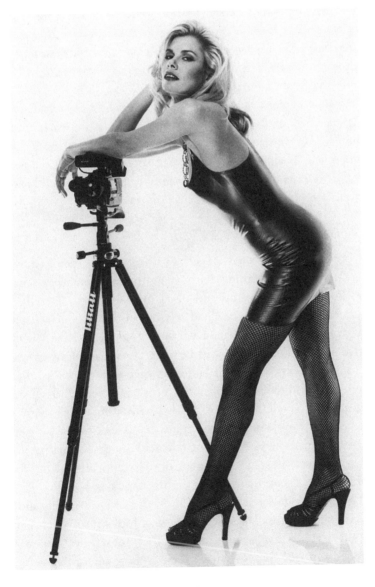

Candida Royalle, a native New Yorker, comes from a background rich in the arts, with training in art, music, voice, and dance. Her educational background includes the New York High School of Arts and Design, Parson's School of Design, and the City University of New York.

In San Francisco, she became active in the avant-garde theater scene, performing with the infamous Cockettes, the Angels of Light, and the late Divine. She later sang in jazz clubs and classical choruses. It was in San Francisco, in the more liberal 1970s, that Ms. Royalle turned to working in X-rated movies for additional income.

In 1984 she founded Femme Productions to create erotic films from a woman's perspective. Her films promoted positive sexual role modeling and were enjoyed by both men and women. Twelve movies later, the Femme line is now distributed worldwide by PHE Inc., who, in partnership with Royalle, will coproduce three new Femme features each year.

Royalle is a founding board member of Feminists for Free Expression (FFE), a nonprofit anticensorship organization. She is the only maker of "adult" films to have been invited to join the American Association of Sex Educators, Counselors, and Therapists (AASECT). She has addressed many conferences in the United States and abroad and has appeared on many major talk shows. She is currently writing a book on female sexual self-empowerment.

✳✳✳

At a young age I liked to draw. Often I drew naked men and women and created a story behind what was going on. I was very sensually aware, but I didn't fool around until my late teens. I really liked boys, and from an early age I had a strong sense of touch. I remember at thirteen having a friend whom I practiced dance with. Our practice sessions would turn into games in which one of us was the boy; we would slowly run our hands up each other's bodies. It never became genital, but I remember feeling very excited and sensual by the touch and smell. I did not do this with a boy until many years later, because boys were always intent on your breasts or genitals. This experience inspired me to display more sensuality in my movies, to show men what women like. I duplicated that scene in my video *Three Daughters* with two eighteen-year-old girls.

The new video I am working on is *Eyes of Desire*. This movie is more serious than my last ones, because it looks into voyeurism and obsessions. I am exploring the idea that sometimes you can get drawn to someone in a way that becomes more of an obsession than a healthy relationship. This reflects quite a change in my work. My earlier movies were quite safe. I made them "soft" because it was a new arena in which women could explore their fantasies. Now my work has become more explicit, but certainly not in the traditional hard-core sense, like erotic films directed by men.

I think women are ready for more—they like seeing men's erections, they like seeing the lovemaking—but I still don't include those come shots all over the place. The other thing that has changed is the exploration of fantasy and the whole delicious aspect of surrendering into your desires and letting your lover dominate you.

When I was a porn star I enjoyed dressing up and playing roles in front of the camera, but the most difficult part for me was engaging in sex in front of the camera. I am not an exhibitionist; in fact, I am a modest person. I worked in the golden age of porn; for thirty-five-millimeter high-budget films, you had to audition and learn lines. This does not happen anymore. As a young struggling artist it was a way of making a lot of money quickly. I prefer being behind the camera. I love creating the script, shooting it, and being in control of the images. I wish I had worked for someone like me when I was an actress, instead of traditional porn moviemakers. When I audition I look for people who bring character and personality to the role, as well as the ability to let go and explore their own eroticism and sensuality. I don't want people who have done so much formulaic work that they just follow the typical porno rules. Acting in porn is a difficult job because you have to take on a role and act it out—yet you must become erotic while still playing the role.

When I was working as a porn actress, if the director and producer were sleazy and didn't really care what they were doing, it made me feel cheap about my profession. But when they took an interest and were creative and innovative, it made me feel good and I was able to give more to the role. I approach my actresses and actors in the way I liked to be approached as an actress. I am very serious about what I do, and I want us to enjoy ourselves as well as to produce a product we all can feel proud of. I expect a lot of professionalism from them, and in return I give them a comfortable and respectful set to work in. I like creating a positive environment for people to work in, and I treat them with a lot of respect, because they are making themselves very vulnerable.

When I can, I always use real-life couples because they add a certain amount of heat. My second choice is to find people who are really hot for one another. I look for chemistry between people.

Safer sex practices and condoms were introduced into my movies in 1987. *Taste of Ambrosia* includes a very sexy scene of a woman putting a black condom on her partner. In *Sensual Escapes* we deal with how to bring up the subject of safe sex. I also feature a safe-sex message at the end of the videos.

I envision erotic films in the future becoming even more of a blend of what women and men are looking for as we grow together. I have started a trend of showing more of what women want sexually and of depicting more sensuality in the sex. Showing the build-up is important, as is the story line. Men watching these movies pay attention to what women like and respond to them and enjoy the experience at the same time. As women grow more comfortable watching these movies, they become open to seeing things that are more racy or explicit.

To maintain excitement in relationships we look for fantasy role-play and ideas. This is reflected in adult movies. The feedback I receive from men who watch my videos is that they love seeing their wives getting excited, which turns them on. Many men tell me they don't like hard-core porn but find my videos very sensual. Women get ideas from the videos to take into their own lives. A young woman who watched my videos told me they opened a new area of possibilities for her. She had been in a relationship for four years that was not very experimental or communicative. Through the inspiration she received from my videos, she was able to try out new things, which were great hits. She learned these new techniques from watching the movies, not by being promiscuous, and this made her feel comfortable about her desires.

Over the years I have done dance, yoga, calisthenics, and weightlifting. These activities enable me to clear my mind. The script for *Eyes of Desire* came from my working out and wondering if anyone could see me. I adapted this into a story of a woman with a high-powered telescope. The twist is that not only does she start getting curious about observing others, but she herself is being observed.

Fantasies are a reflection of what is happening in our life. For myself, running my own company, I have to constantly be in a powerful position, and there is nothing more delicious than giving up that control. Also, I believe that the basis of our fantasies comes from our upbringing and how sexuality was presented to us when we were growing up. I come from a Catholic background where sex was forbidden—you had to save yourself. For a lot of women this has instilled a sense of shame and guilt about our sexuality. Therefore, to lose control and have an orgasm and receive pleasure, we have to pretend we are being forced to give up that control. This is what gives rise to the "rape" fantasy; we obviously don't want to be raped in real life, but we need a trigger that gives us permission to receive pleasure and give up control.

A wonderful, sexy thing to do in a relationship is to write your fantasy to your lover and leave it in a secret note, or read to him or her a story from an erotic novel. Once you have shared your fantasies, there is nothing sexier than to speak your partner's favorite fantasy out loud while your partner pleasures himself or herself or while you pleasure your partner. Fantasy is not necessarily something you act out. I was in a monogamous relationship where we would fantasize about the other being with someone else, but in real life we were very possessive and jealous. However, we would talk about it and make believe, which was very positive for us and a great way to play.

Exercise: Thoughts on Making Your Own Home Movies

Watching movies opens you up, gives you ideas, and gets you in touch with inner fantasies that you might not have been aware of. Self-pleasuring as you watch erotic videos is a very good way to feel connected with your fantasies without judging them.

Making your own home movies can be sexy and fun, but I believe couples should put a lot of thought into whether it's a good idea for them. There is always the possibility that the video will be found and circulated. Because I am now a very private person, I never let myself be photographed or videotaped in a sexual situation.

One way to have the fun of making your own erotic home movie without actually recording a videotape is to use a video camera without any film. Hook the camcorder up to a TV monitor, and watch yourself and your partner making love on TV. This can be very exciting.

NAN KINNEY

Pornography: Expanding Our Sexual Horizons

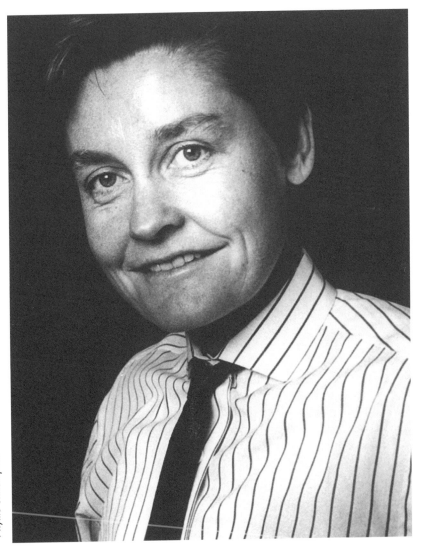

Phyllis Christopher

Nan Kinney is the producer of Fatale videos and one of the founding publishers of the highly acclaimed and notorious magazine On Our Backs. *A native of Austin, Minnesota, she began her foray into the world of lesbian pornography in the early 1980s when she moved to San Francisco to check out the SM scene.*

When she realized there was no venue for lesbian sexual imagery made by and for lesbians, she and two partners, Deborah Sundahl and Susie Bright, solicited material and published their first issue of On Our Backs *in June 1984. With the success and popularity of the magazine, Nan and Deborah jumped into videos.*

In January 1985, they released Private Pleasures *and* Shadows, *two videos that starred real-life lesbian lovers and presented for the first time sexually explicit footage made by and for lesbians. Later titles included* Suburban Dykes, Safe Is Desire, How to Female Ejaculate, Hungry Hearts, *and* Burlezk Live I *and* II.

By 1994, with On Our Backs *being published bimonthly and the circulation at an all-time high, Nan and Deborah decided to sell the magazine and pursue their separate interests.*

Nan now runs Fatale Videos full-time and has expanded the company's mission to include bisexual pornographic images. A recent release, Bend Over Boyfriend, *starring sex educators Carol Queen and Robert Morgan, addresses women giving men anal pleasure. Currently in production is* Rev Her Up, *a fun-filled lesbian urban romp through the back rooms of an auto-repair shop.*

Nan's goal has always been to present alternative images of sexuality, and she has now expanded the goal to include bisexual images. She believes that sex is an important part of people's lives and that women—lesbians in particular—have always been portrayed in a very limited way in traditional pornography. She wants people to have other images of themselves as a way to burst out of the ingrained images in mainstream porn.

✳✳✳

The inspiration for *On Our Backs* came from the fact that there was no porn for lesbians. We went to a bookshop, trying to find some porn, and all we found was one book. I wanted more. They didn't even have *The Story of O.* I always liked pornography; I always liked to read *Playboy* and *Penthouse,* and I wanted something authentic, a magazine made by and for lesbians. I wanted to produce something that more realistically represented my sexuality as a butch lesbian.

I wasn't alone in this desire for sexually explicit images of lesbians. All my friends were taking pictures of one another and didn't have a place to publish them. We knew there was a need. We wanted it, so we figured other people wanted it too. This was in 1984, the time of the sex wars in the lesbian community, when lesbians were marching at the frontlines of the antiporn movement with Andrea Dworkin and Catherine MacKinnon.

On the flip side were these sexually active, radical lesbians who thought sex was great and pornography was a viable way to explore our sexuality together, to expand our sexual horizons. Obviously, I was part of the latter group. We did it as sort of a political move in the beginning rather than a business move. It was a great way of fighting back at the antiporn feminists and of making a statement for pro-sex lesbians, many of whom also considered themselves feminists.

I literally had been in bed with women who wouldn't let me penetrate them because it wasn't politically correct. It pissed me off that the feminist political bullshit had infiltrated these women's sex lives. They were denying themselves pleasure because of it. It also was a very special time in San Francisco in 1984, a creative time. Politics was the glue that brought us together. We wanted to make our mark on the world.

The lesbian community's reaction to the first issue of *On Our Backs* was totally overwhelming—either for or against—a very strong reaction. We got hate mail. We got people in our faces calling us Nazis at San Francisco's Gay Pride celebration, where we had a booth. But it was more overwhelmingly positive than negative. "Thank God!" they'd say. "Finally something I can relate to and get off on!" We got enough support to publish more issues. People sent us submissions for the magazine—erotic stories and pictures came pouring in from all over the country.

Some of the artists and writers were already established, such as Tee Corrine, Lee Lynch, Joan Nestle, Dorothy Allison, Pat Califia. Others essentially started their erotic publishing careers with *On Our Backs*, for instance photographers Morgan Gwenwald, Honey Lee Cotrell, Phyllis Christopher, and Jill Posner and fiction writers such as Jewell Gomez.

Because *On Our Backs* got such attention, we realized there were other ways to produce porn. It was natural. We wanted to be the Mitchell Brothers of the lesbian porn world. (The Mitchell Brothers are the owners of the well-known San Francisco O'Farrell

Theater, a strip club, and producers of videos.) It was fun! We had a great time. We also began to make some money.

Women loved it. The women-only strip show *Burlezk* ran sold-out weekly shows for four years. At that time no distributors existed for the types of videos we made; we had to sell them ourselves through direct mail and advertising in *On Our Backs*. Once again, response was overwhelming. Our mailbag was full every day. We'd get letters that were very explicit from readers and viewers. They'd say, "I want to see more hairy butches," or "Thanks for your images of big women. Let's see more." So we knew we were on the right track.

Now I'm strictly in the video business and focusing on producing and selling Fatale videos. There are more distributors now that will carry the videos. I'm thinking of Good Vibrations in particular, but also of lesbian- and gay-friendly video companies around the country. I've expanded the subject matter to include bisexual women's points of view, because there is nothing really made for them either. You can find videos with two guys and a girl, but that's not the same. Our latest release is *Bend Over Boyfriend*, an informative tape about how to pleasure your man anally, which I believe is the first of its kind. It's selling like mad and has frequently been the number one best-selling video for Good Vibrations. This tells me there is a need for this type of imagery.

My life really hasn't changed because of that era. I'm the same person. I'm still a lesbian pornographer, which is what I always wanted to be when I grew up. One of my biggest role models was Larry Flynt. Also Hugh Hefner, the Mitchell Brothers, Gloria Steinem, Joani Blank (founder of Good Vibrations)—these people were my role models. I'm still following the goals I had at that time.

I've always seen myself on the outside of things culturally, sexually, politically. I'm a daredevil. I don't have any preconceived notions of how my life should be. I'm willing to try different things. In the 1980s I explored SM because at that time those were the only lesbians talking about sex. Or even practicing it, doing it. I was curious, and I had the opportunity to explore it, but I learned it doesn't get me off that much. I learned it's not SM I'm into as much as being open to sex in general, to my sexuality around butch and femme, that sort of thing.

I'm the same person sexually that I was in high school, but I'm more at ease with myself now. I'm a Taurus; I'm a butch who likes femmes. I've explored a lot of things, but I've come back to the fact that this is what my sexuality is. I'm your basic meat-and-potatoes butch. I like a girlfriend; I like a house; I like my work. I'm not that different from most people. It's just that my work is producing sexual images, which puts me outside the American mainstream. Also, I have had the bonus of having better sex because of my job.

I want more of the same for the future—back to the future, if you will. For as long as I'm able, I want to be a producer of pornography. I'd like to be able to bring somebody up in the business and let them have it. I want to encourage young women coming into the porn business, to be a mentor of young women, of lesbians in particular.

Presently, my video *Rev Her Up* is in the works. I'm trying for the first time to put humor and sex together. Can people really laugh when they have sex? When they're turned on? Does laughter turn them on? I have a gut feeling from all the times I've laughed in bed that we can hit that spot with a video. Having just relocated to New York, I've put together a different team of women and men to work on this film. Even though it will be a lesbian video, we'll have men in minor roles because men—gay men especially—are in our lives.

The other thing we're doing is exploring international sales and distribution of all our titles. We still encounter difficulty in some countries with censorship. This is an age-old issue. From the start of my career, fighting censorship has been part of my job, part of the essential work I have to do. In the beginning it was censorship within the lesbian community, and now I'm dealing with censorship on an international level.

The Internet offers a potential solution to some of this, but you still have to mail your product into foreign countries, and the stores cannot display it. Even in New York City this is happening, under the mayor's plan to turn the city into one big Disneyworld. On the Internet, however, we can display our products. The Internet is a great frontier, although we don't know how it's going to turn out, especially with pending American legislation that would limit what's available on the Internet.

Tips: Roses, Vodka, and Videotape— How to Watch a Porn Movie

As with any sort of sexual foreplay, watching dirty movies together with your partner doesn't always work. You usually can't just pick one off the shelf, pop it in the VCR, sit back, and expect to get horny. (Unless, of course, you're already horny and the video is really just the signal to make love, like adjusting the lighting or putting on some sexy music.) Using porn videos as foreplay takes some forethought. Here's my advice on the subject.

Assuming you're looking to a porn video as part of the seduction or turn-on, I find the biggest pitfall is expecting too much from an erotic or porn video. People who haven't watched a lot of porn are often surprised and disappointed at the low production quality, poor scripts, bad acting, and the general formulaic, juvenile, and male-oriented content. This disappointment can be a true turn-off. So the most important thing I have to say about watching porn is: be forgiving.

Try to find one thing in a video that turns you on. If you can find even that one thing, I think the video is a success. Maybe it's a certain camera angle that lets you see what it looks like from your partner's point of view when she's fucking you. Maybe it's a look in one of the actress's eyes, a stance, a sentence, an orgasmic scream, anything that sends a twitch to your clit and that you can hold onto for later fantasies.

Learning how to appreciate porn can take time. Be patient. Do it with your partner. Rent a lot of tapes until you find the ones that arouse you, and think about what you like about it so you can home in on the types of porn you should be getting. Talk about it with your partner—maybe you'll find you like different sorts of porn. For example, I think of porn videos like I think of action movies: some sort of plot is needed, but it's really all about the action, the sex. I have my favorite action heroes (Arnold Schwarzenegger, Linda Hamilton) and I have my favorite porn heroes (Sharon Mitchell, Nina Hartley). Usually I can watch anything they do and get into it.

So once you've found some porn you like, make an evening of it! Have a video date—buy your honey some roses, have a little vodka (or a beverage of your choice), wear something you feel sexy in. Bring out your collection of porn videos, or get something new (but within your predeter- mined rating of the potential for turn-on). Get comfort- able—no phones, no kids, no neighbors. Let the tape roll and the juices will flow.

Sex Positivism

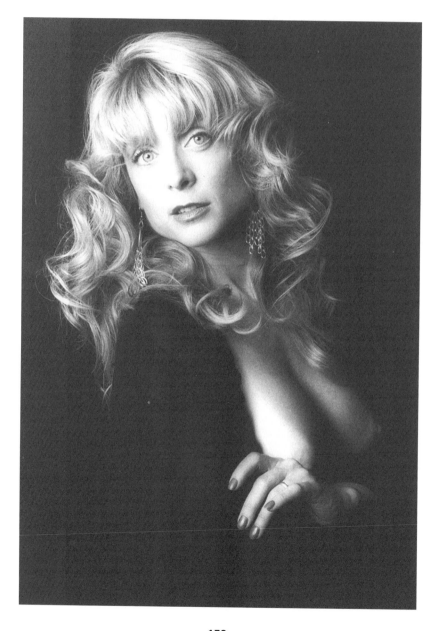

Nina Hartley, R.N., is a fifteen-year veteran of "adult" videos. She is a dancer, educator, director, actress, advocate, activist, writer, and swinger. One of the most vocal of the sex-positive feminists who came on the scene in the mid-1980s, she is tireless in promoting her sexual philosophy, a unique synthesis of science, humanism, feminism, socialism, and personal responsibility. A charismatic and engaging speaker, she is popular with a wide range of audiences.

After starting as a dancer while going to nursing school in California, Nina found she liked the explicit medium of film well enough to make the transition. In 1985, after graduating magna cum laude, she went full-time into the movies. She has been the winner of most of the porn industry's most prestigious awards, and she continues to act, as well as produce, direct, and write her own videos. She lives with her husband, Dave, and her wife, Bobby, in a longstanding ménage à trois in Berkeley, California.

✳✳✳

I was one of the first women to declare myself a feminist porn star, and the title now represents my abiding love of women (and by extension, men) in all its manifestations. It obligates me to engage the world, to share my knowledge with interested people, and to champion the cause of sex positivism in an otherwise hostile environment. It is because of my passionate sex-positive feminism that I find the energy to engage "the enemy" in dialogue rather than shut them out. It is a statement of self-love that does not come at the expense of others; instead, it is at the service of others.

Initially, I publicly identified as a feminist because I believed in the principles of gender equality and wanted to promote them. I wanted to bring a feminist eye to the inner workings of commercial pornography, not just read theoretical treatises on the evils of objectification. If sexual self-determination was every woman's birthright and if my body was truly mine, then I concluded there was no reason why I could not conduct myself with feminist-inspired self-respect within the world of sex work.

Frankly, I also did it to make myself more interesting to journalists and scholars and to lead them in my direction as someone who was willing to speak to them. At the time, I was one of the few performers who were willing to talk to "outsiders" about the business. Although feminists were talking about porn, few were talking to the people who made it. Fewer still were involved in making it.

In general, feminists felt themselves better than "those women" who were willing to subjugate themselves to such an exploitative industry. Their arrogance permitted them to ignore sex workers' stories and summarily dismiss what they had to say. Well, I was of their class and educational background, so they were unable to dismiss me easily. I wanted to be an articulate defender of sexually oriented material and of consensual sexual behavior, no matter how "kinky" it seemed to the uninitiated.

I try to keep my family life separate from my work. My husband is intensely private, and I honor that. My wife, Bobby, and I would have more of an open-door policy with regard to friends and the media. Out of respect for his sensibilities, however, we limit the people we allow into our home. Instead, we go to their place. There are certain topics that are not totally open for discussion during interviews. Because my public persona is very closely aligned with my "real" self, there is very little problem for me in making the transition from "in public" to "at home."

I tend to form relationships with other sex-positive people: we all love to talk shop! The discussions we have are very exciting. With fans, I expect a lot of sexual talk, but I don't normally discuss any trials and tribulations with them. I love any opportunity to share my sexual journey with interested viewers or readers. As a self-identified, out exhibitionist, the satisfactory expression of my sexuality depends in part on its being public, that is, enjoyed by others as entertainment or education. When it comes to my most deeply personal emotional experiences, I must first experience them in private before I can think of translating them to the screen or stage.

I am now fifteen years into my career, and I produce, direct, and star in a successful line of sex education videos, from which I receive a royalty (one of the first performers to do so). I am starting to make inroads into "straight" projects, most notably a part in the 1997 film *Boogie Nights*. I'm increasing my profile as a lecturer, advocate, educator, and pundit, in addition to "merely" being an entertainer. As always, I mentor novice performers and provide a sympathetic ear for people with sexual problems.

My work has changed as I've matured and become more experienced as a performer. What has remained the same is my dedication to showcasing empowered, positive, female sexuality. I've always tried to be an accessible role model for women who are developing their own sexual identities. Now I just have a bigger venue for it.

I see myself working as an actress for as long as I want. As the boomers age, they (especially the women) desire and deserve to see themselves represented onscreen as viable, sexy people. Performers my age can only benefit from this unique demographic phenomenon. Fans tend to be fans for life: if nothing else, their adoration alone will guarantee a livelihood of sorts for me as long as I wish to continue. As I grow and change, my fans are interested in hearing about it and, if at all possible, seeing it for themselves. The nature of my representation may change, but it will continue to be made available to those who desire it.

I see my career going in a direction that befits an older woman and crone-in-training: education, advocacy, and sexual mastery. I have become a valuable resource to the community and for those who will come after me. I hope I will always have younger people around me to draw inspiration from and to inspire in return. That exchange of energy and ideas propels the culture forward.

I have had the rare experience of having had significantly more and varied sexual partners than the average person. My training as a health professional, combined with my exhibitionism and feminist perspective, has given me a unique insight into a very complex issue. Some fundamental truths: men are just as sexually oppressed as women, only in different areas; men need tenderness and caring and touching just as much as women (in fact, they are starved for it); women who share their sexuality with kindness as opposed to vindictiveness wield tremendous power; men will follow our rules if we will only articulate them; most men want to see women sexually happy—all they want to do is join in and be a part of the process; men in the grip of sexual arousal and desire are often at their sweetest and most accessible and are easily guided.

I've learned that sexuality is very fluid and that lines blur (especially in the presence of an experienced partner) with little effort. I've come to appreciate the power of sexual arousal and ecstasy to transform people, to heal their spirits, to radically alter their consciousness permanently and for the better. Sexual contact reaches into the depths of a person, transmitting more information in a single moment than can be communicated any other way.

I've learned that the directness of the sexual experience transcends language barriers, that it truly is the international language. Touch is the ultimate and primal universal communication. I've learned that sexual skills can be taught and passed on, like any other skills, for the betterment of the participants.

Currently, bringing women into the sex industry as consumers is very important to me. I want to contribute to a body of work that speaks to their sexuality as opposed to only trying to capture the "average" male's interest. I want to educate women and empower them to honor their sexuality, for it can save the world. I want to expand the range of sexually explicit material to encompass more varied sexual interests. I want to promote women's control of reproduction. The issue of the dominant culture's attitude toward and treatment of my chosen profession (and, by extension, of my sexuality itself) is one I love to address. Taking my sex-positive message to the greater society is very compelling to me.

Exercise: How to Create a Porn Fantasy at Home

All we professionals do onscreen is to playact the scripts given to us or, if it's an amateur video, the scripts we give ourselves. It's just role-playing around a basic premise or scenario.

To role-play a porn fantasy at home, each of you must first pick or create a character that excites you. Then decide what kind of energy you'll be playing with. Next, you'll need to decide on the setting, that is, the location and situation. You may want to negotiate the type of sex ahead of time, for example, rape, seduction, love fucking, sport fucking, a blow job, or mutual masturbation.

Next, put on costumes (if you want to) and start role-playing. Go ahead and act out the role you've chosen. This is the ultimate in improvisational theater. The idea is to have fun and develop intimacy. If it stops being fun, stop the activity. Keep it up for as long as you feel like it. That's all it takes to make your own porn "movie."

PART 9

Women's Sex Shops

In 1962 Beate Uhse opened the first sex shop in the world, the Sex Institute of Marital Hygiene in Flensburg, Germany. She later opened similar shops in other German cities and became a notorious celebrity in the process. She also set up porn theaters to show what were then known as "blue" movies—but the market for her adult businesses was most definitely men.

Eve's Garden, established by Dell Williams in 1973 as a mail-order business based in New York City, was the world's first sex shop targeting women customers. The impetus for it came out of the first Women's Sexuality Conference in New York and from Dell's friendship with Betty Dodson, who was leading masturbation workshops for women.

Dell started her business with two products and ran the operation from her home. As the business grew, she developed the product range and in 1978 opened a retail shop on Manhattan's Upper East Side. Her main product lines were books and vibrators, which she hoped would educate women about how to have orgasms. This was a major move from the traditional sex-shop approach, where so much about sexuality was left unsaid and the main emphasis was on lingerie to create a sexual atmosphere. Dell was a pro-sex feminist who believed in women's liberation without religious or political interference.

In 1977 Joani Blank opened Good Vibrations in San Francisco, which encompassed both a mail-order catalogue and a retail shop. It was very different from Xandria and Adam and Eve, the other contemporary mail-order businesses, both based in San Francisco, which centered on men's sexual products and needs. The pro-sex environment of Good Vibrations focused on offering quality vibrators and videos for women, whether lesbian, bisexual, or heterosexual.

In the early 1990s Hanni Jagtman and Ellen van der Gang opened Mail and Female in Amsterdam, the first mail-order catalogue for women in Europe. They realized that, even in liberated Amsterdam, many women were not comfortable visiting the existing retail stores. As the business grew, Mail and Female branched out, and locations named Female and Partners were also added in Holland, Belgium, and Spain. Eighty to 90 percent of their customers were women, most over thirty years of age, who wanted to purchase vibrators and clothing to improve their sex lives.

In Australia in the early 1990s no sex shops existed that were designed for women. Existing sex shops were based on meeting male's sexual needs and were typified by rows of "girlie" magazines and videos, badly designed phallic-shaped vibrators and dildos, with a man (who frequently knew nothing of female sexuality) behind the counter. The atmosphere was sleazy, and most women who entered the environment felt embarrassed.

Courses in the area of sex-positive sexuality were by this time being offered in Australia, however, and a natural progression led in 1992 to my opening the Pleasure Spot. It was the first mail-order catalogue to focus on what women wanted (a retail shop was added later in Sydney). The design and layout of the catalogues made it easy for women to purchase from them, as they included descriptions of how and why to use each product. The main emphasis was on a female-oriented, sensual, uninhibited yet respectable marketing approach. New products, inspired by those available in the United States, were designed, including silicon dildos shaped as whales, dolphins, goddesses, and intertwined lovers; plug-in vibrators and videos featuring helpful sex education; female erotica; and sensual products. Courses were available to support women and couples on their sexual journey.

The Pleasure Spot's new and different style made competing with the traditional sex outlets difficult. The older, well-established businesses had large budgets for marketing and advertising, while the Pleasure Spot relied on an up-front media profile for its sex-positive approach. Thousands and thousands of women and their partners responded enthusiastically to this new way of looking at sexuality.

Recently, in Japan, Minori Kitahara rejected the traditional male-dominated Japanese culture she had been brought up in to bravely introduce a new type of sexuality to Japanese women. She followed the trailblazing women in the West by starting the women's sex shop Love Piece and its accompanying mail-order catalogue.

Ky began Sh! in 1992 in London after being frustrated in her attempts to find basic female sexual products. She felt women's needs were not being addressed in the existing male-owned and -run shops. The response to her new business was fantastic, reflecting what had happened in the United States, Holland, Japan, and Australia, where women supported other women in this new approach to feminist sexuality.

JO-ANNE BAKER

Putting Sexuality in the Right Perspective

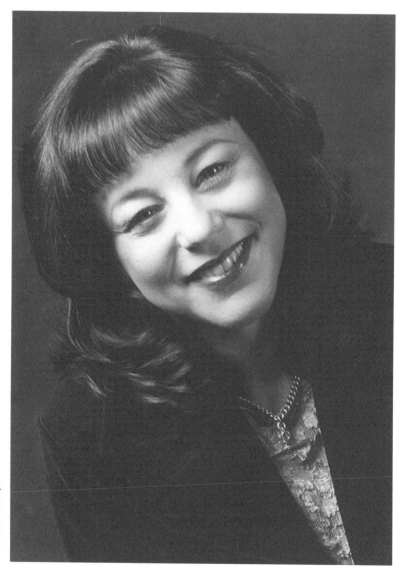

Matthew Scroope

Jo-Anne Baker has worked in the area of sexuality since 1990. Her business, the

Pleasure Spot, was the first in Australia to focus on women's and couples' sexuality. It introduced a wide variety of sex toys, videos, and literature that previously had been unavailable, as well as courses on spiritual and sexual growth.

After receiving her sociology degree, Jo-Anne traveled widely. She lived in the U.K., the United States, and Italy, where she trained in erotic spirituality. This included studying bioenergetics, hypnotherapy, meditation, Tantra, sex positivism, macrobiotics, astrology, and massage. She successfully introduced futons to Australia in the 1980s, revolutionizing the bedding market.

She is well-known as one of Australia's leading sex entrepreneurs, counselors, and educators, and articles about her work have appeared in national magazines and newspapers, and on TV and radio. Jo-Anne now focuses on her writing and sexual counseling. Her previous book is Self-Sexual Healing: Finding Pleasure Within.

❋❋❋

My quest to understand my own sexuality did not start until the 1980s, when I participated in many self-development courses and workshops that focused on learning how to connect with my body and expand my sensuality. I wanted to heal the sexual repression I had grown up with and learn how to be relaxed with myself.

My journey to find sexual fulfillment took me around the globe, visiting women who have changed history by bringing sexual taboos out of the darkness, and teaching women how to experience pleasure, fun, and lots of sexual fulfillment. There is never enough time to explore the depths of pleasure and sensuality that are possible for each one of us.

In 1992 I started the Pleasure Spot, an adjunct to the courses on sexuality I was organizing. It was at first a mail-order business and later became the first retail sex shop for women in Australia. I felt it was essential to put sexuality in the right perspective, to remove the connotations that sex was dirty, bad, or something to be ashamed of. Many sex products and all but a few sex shops had been designed by men, who believed they knew what women wanted. For many women, this was far from true. I visited the existing women's sex shops around the world, including Eve's Garden in New York, Good Vibrations in San Francisco, Sh! in London, Mail and Female in Amsterdam—and all of them inspired me with their innovative approach to sexuality.

When I set up the business I paid special attention to sensual products—such as feathers, candles, edible oils, and powders—as well as nonphallic dildos. I stocked plug-in vibrators, which were then a novelty in Australia, and they quickly caught on.

I sold products and ran and organized courses designed to teach women how to feel more relaxed and alive in their bodies. The courses included breath and energy orgasms, striptease, and erotic massage. They became popular with men, too, so I included evenings for couples and for men only.

Many women are still embarrassed to visit a sex shop and to talk about sexuality, because they feel that the area is taboo or they have feelings of shame about their body or their erotic desires. Thousands of women have begun conversations with me at the Pleasure Spot with, "I have never told anyone about this" or "I feel really embarrassed to ask you about this" or "I am probably the only one to feel this way" or "Is there something wrong with me because I like. . . ." I have found that men and women are desperate for clear, accurate sexual information that is free of judgment, sleaze, and double entendres.

Overwhelmingly, the issues my clients want to discuss do not surprise me, and I have been able to reassure them that their sexual desires or interests are not only "normal," but healthy. We live in such a sex-negative culture that any positive information on sexuality and the human body is still desperately sought. It is amazing that since the 1960s we have been able to go to the moon, yet at the turn of the century so many people are still divorced from the body they live in. We all exist because a sexual act created us, and to be at emotional and physical peace we need to learn to embrace our sexuality.

Since 1990 thousands of Australians have contacted me for products and advice. Doctors and therapists started sending clients with sexual difficulties to me. This encouraged me to develop my own form of body-orientated sexual-healing sessions and eventually to publish *Self-Sexual Healing: Finding Pleasure Within*, a step-by-step guide to healing, with practical exercises and techniques.

Exercise: The Wave

(From *Self-Sexual Healing: Finding Pleasure Within*, exercise 2.6)

Time: Ten to fifteen minutes

Setting: A room where you will not be disturbed, or out in
nature

Music: Something sensual, with a repeated melody

Lighting: Natural or candles

I have worked with many people to help them feel more
connected to their bodies. This is a simple exercise to
accomplish that by helping you relax and expand your
physical flexibility. When you feel relaxed with the movement you can take it into lovemaking and masturbation.
An added advantage is that it is good for your back!

When a woman gives birth her body undulates like a wave.
This movement is also repeated in a woman's orgasm—a
ripple effect goes through the body. For men this movement helps the pelvis relax into a backward and forward
motion, rather than the traditional sensations, which are
like a band of sexual tension that builds up to ejaculation.
The wave exercise deliberately exaggerates the natural sexual movement, teaching you a wonderful way to turn yourself on and pulse the sexual energy throughout the body.

To begin, lie down on the floor with your knees bent.
Place one of your palms of your hand on the top of your
head and start to move your pelvis backward and forward
in a gentle rocking motion. Do not take your bottom off
the ground. You will find if you are doing the movement
correctly that the top of your head moves, your back
arches, and your lower back remains on the floor. If you
take your bottom off the floor, you will find you will put
pressure on your lower back. If done correctly, this exercise
also helps bad back problems.

Connect with the sensations as you move your body,
becoming conscious of how your head moves. It is very

common for people to feel movement only in the pelvis and not in the spine or head. If that happens, try again, exaggerating the pelvis's backward and forward motion so that both the top of your head and your spine also start to move.

Allow your inhalation to become stronger, as if you were breathing through a straw; let your exhalation happen naturally. Incorporate your breath with the movement: on the inhalation, clench your pelvic-floor muscles (which are the muscles you use to stop yourself from urinating), and relax on the exhalation. To enable more relaxation, imagine your pelvis falling, as though into quicksand, as you exhale. Once you have mastered this movement you can remove your hand, as it is only there to help guide you in moving your whole body.

As you find your own natural rhythm, try visualizing light moving in waves from your genitals up through the body to the top of your head. Let any sound be expressed, especially if you visualize color or movement in the throat area. You can also incorporate using a vibrator into the exercise. The main focuses are on expanding the senses, moving the sexual energy throughout the body, and being turned on.

This exercise can become the foundation to help you connect with feelings of sensuality and expand your eroticism with a partner by moving and breathing.

Talking Sex

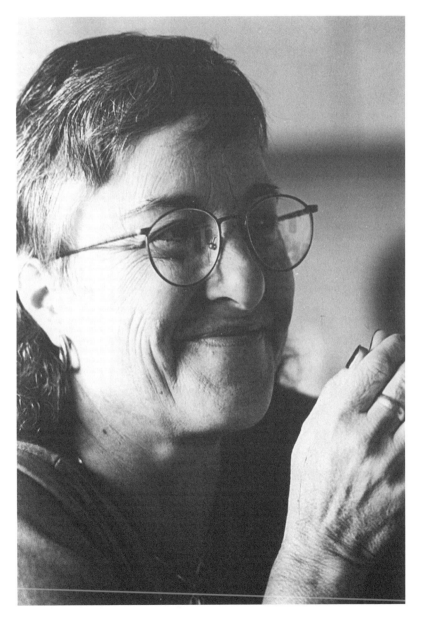

Joani Blank was born in 1937 and raised in Boston. She holds a master's degree in public health education, with a special interest in family planning. In the mid-1960s she believed she was headed for a career in international family planning.

When Joani moved to San Francisco in 1971, she realized that sex was a much more intriguing field of inquiry than birth control, although the two fields are obviously related. Joani's realization that women's difficulties with contraception were connected with their discomfort with their sexuality changed the direction of her life's work.

Joani is renowned as the founder of Good Vibrations, San Francisco's famous sex toy, book, and video store and mail-order service, which opened in 1977. Long dedicated to democratic business management, in 1992 she converted Good Vibrations into a worker cooperative; it is now wholly owned by its employees, of which she is no longer one.

She formed Down There Press, Good Vibrations' sister publishing company, in 1975. She is author or editor of eight of the fifteen titles currently published by Down There Press. Her books include Good Vibrations, I Am My Lover, A Kid's First Book About Sex, First Person Sexual, Femalia, *and the forthcoming* Still Doing It. *In 1996, Joani, doing business as Blank Tapes, produced and directed two videos,* Carol Queen's Great Vibrations *and* Faces of Ecstasy.

Joani has a lot of interests that have nothing to do with sex. One of these is cohousing, a form of cooperative housing that originated in Denmark and is spreading with deliberate speed in North America, where close to fifty cohousing communities are now built and occupied. She sings in a choir, is learning Taiko drumming, is engaged in socially responsible investing, and does volunteer work.

She is a mother and grandmother and would like to be a little less single than she is at present, but she's not quite sure if monogamy works for her.

✳✳✳

Dell Williams' business, Eve's Garden, was one of my earliest inspirations. Her business was mail-order, but I wanted to open a retail store. My concept was to have a store where people could touch, hold, and feel sex toys and be able to have long conversations with staff about the different products. In 1977 I opened the door to my San Francisco shop, Good Vibrations. My staff are all sex educators, and it has always been important to me that they receive very good training. Good Vibrations has had 150,000 customers, both male and female, since it opened.

What happened during the 1970s in Western society had very little to do with the sexual act itself, but it had to do with the ability of women to control their fertility, via the birth control pill. The Pill basically led to women's liberation. Without the Pill it is unlikely that the women's liberation of the 1970s would have happened with the speed it did. In terms of the sexual revolution, nowadays it is very unlikely that a woman would grow into adulthood without knowing where her clitoris is and what it is for. This is very different from when I was growing up.

On some levels things have changed, but in many quarters our society is actually going backward with regard to sex education, now that schools have introduced Christian-based, abstinence-only sex education programs. These have proven not to work in terms of preventing STDs (sexually transmitted diseases) and teenage pregnancies. Sexual repression is worse because the radical right has promoted so much negativity and ignorance about sex. In the process, a generation of kids are being created who, when they do get around to having sex, are going to hate it.

It is my contention that the worst sexual dysfunction we have as a society is our inability to talk about sex. The thing that interests me the most, and what I like to do in workshops, is to find ways for people to talk about sex. If we could treat sex as just one of a range of things that people do, instead of something special that belongs over there, separate from everything else, we could create a whole different atmosphere around sex. It would be easier to talk about sex, to bring it up in conversation and acknowledge a sexual attraction between people.

Instead, we've alienated sex from the rest of our lives. Sex, in fact, is not separate from the rest of our lives. I decided recently that psychoanalyst Sigmund Freud was right when he said that at some level everything is about sex. The fact that we put sex aside to make it something special creates an amazing amount of anxiety around all aspects of sexuality. It's problematic, because if you say, "Let's get rid of all the anxiety around sex," then you get rid of a lot of the excitement, too. I do not have a particularly spiritual orientation toward sexuality. However, as I get older I can see that the root of our sexual issues—for example, the things that excite us, freak us out, embarrass us, and make us anxious—are all reflections of what happens in our everyday life.

I lead a variety of sex workshops where I encourage people to communicate more openly. In my women's workshops, they learn to be more assertive, to show their sexual strengths as opposed to weaknesses, to get to the point where they believe they deserve to receive pleasure, whatever that takes. A woman can learn what she wants sexually through masturbation; she then needs to learn how to honestly convey that to her partner.

In the men's workshops, they explore being vulnerable by expressing what they are feeling. In one such workshop, a man told me that he had difficulty forming sexual relationships. I told him that the most important thing was to be vulnerable with his partner. He needed to learn to say, "I've been out on four dates with you, and I am scared to hold your hand." It is so powerful to say to someone what you are truly experiencing.

I also run a group workshop called *How to Get What You Want in Bed or Wherever Else You Do It.* As part of this workshop, the group has an open discussion about the various reasons why they have difficulty asserting themselves sexually and asking for what they want. I have found that many people focus on their fear of rejection. In this workshop we face the fear by getting people to ask for what they want—and then getting rejected. We do this with an emphasis on fun; I encourage a lot of laughter. People also have to be able to say, "No, I don't want to." It's been a very powerful exercise for people, because it gets the couples talking about sex.

I did this workshop recently at a Unitarian church retreat for about fifteen people, made up of couples and singles of all sexual orientations. After the course, people opened up and started talking about sex, asking one another about the most interesting places they had masturbated. The participants in the workshop found that you can talk about sex and that it is good. You learn about other people and realize that you are not weird and that you are not a terrible person.

My message is to do it! Find fun, creative ways to get what you want in bed by deciding who initiates sex, who does what when, what kind of games you like to play. Use basic assertiveness techniques. Many people can't imagine that there is any way to talk about sex unless they are in bed, which is not the case. It is important to talk about sex at a nonsexual time. You can also write letters to one another about what you like physically, but make sure it is an

equal commitment. In many heterosexual relationships it is often
the woman who perceives that she is not getting what she wants
from her male partner, while men want to "fix" their female partners. I tell them to focus on changing themselves first. It does not
help a woman to feel as if she is a "patient" who has to be "cured"
of her "problem."

Very few people get as much sex as they like or the kind of sex
they want. There are also many people who have lots of sex but are
not sexually satisfied. I want to help people change that for themselves! I am in my sixties and I am more sexually active and positive
than I have ever been in my life.

Tip: How to Have a Better Orgasm

If you are doing all the right things but still having difficulty coming, here's a tip that works well for me. First,
decide how aroused you are on a scale from one to ten,
with ten being the most aroused. Do not change the stimulation, but pay attention to how warm you are, the
amount of tension you have in your legs, and what you are
experiencing in your body. This includes how genitally
turned-on you feel. Then try to intentionally lower the
number you have decided on.

For example, if you decide that your level of arousal is at
an eight, try to intentionally bring your level of arousal to
a lower level without changing the level of stimulation you
are receiving. Try to make yourself less aroused. This is a
paradoxical instruction. When you tell yourself to be less
aroused by trying to lower the number on your scale of
arousal, the opposite naturally occurs, and you become
more excited.

Tune In to Your True Erotic Nature

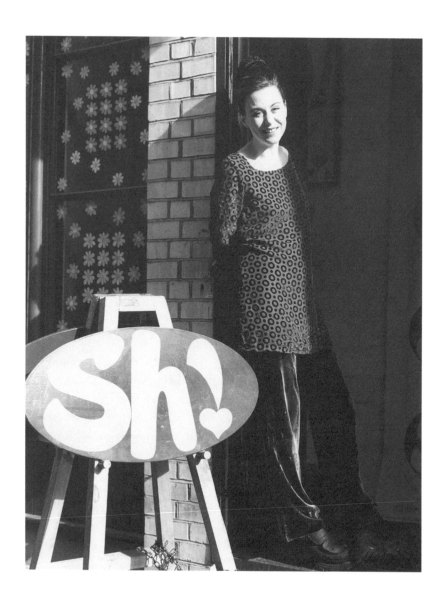

Ky is originally from Yorkshire, U.K. After leaving school she studied at art school and earned a degree in alternative practice. In her words, she "pratted around," which included periods of being unemployed, stints as a nanny, and working in Japan teaching English. She is the proprietor of Sh!, a women's erotic emporium in London.

❋❋❋

The inspiration for Sh! started in 1992, when I went shopping with a close friend, Kim, to buy a strap-on dildo and harness for her. We started in Soho and then spread our search to the sex shops around London. We started in inner London and moved outward in greater concentric circles until it got ridiculous. We went from shop to shop, amazed that we couldn't find what she wanted.

All the dildos and harnesses were either crappy and badly designed—impractical with no idea of what a woman wanted—or they were made for gay leathermen, leather daddies, with all the dildos in realistic penis shapes. At first we thought this was funny, but soon it became depressing and very demoralizing. I found that at many sex shops, employees were very uncomfortable when we went in, and I got the strong feeling we weren't supposed to be there. If women feel uncomfortable in sex shops, it is because that is how they are made to feel—as though they are polluting the atmosphere with all their estrogen or something. A 1950s atmosphere of "nice girls don't" pervades many of these shops—and I got really cross about it.

At the time, there was a great deal of public sexuality education about AIDS and safe sex. Women were urged to talk about what they wanted sexually, and about the use of condoms and safe sex. I began to wonder what this all meant when women like myself, who considered themselves sexually literate and sexual outlaws, couldn't find what they wanted. What were straighter, more conservative women going to do? How were they coping? It was during our travels around these sex shops that Kim and I started to discuss opening our own shop for women. It started off as a joke, but as we became more and more annoyed, we became more and more serious about it. Kim was an accountant, so she looked into the possibility and thought it was financially feasible. Her encouragement fired me along, but although I was angry at the lack of products for women and believed a market existed for them, I was unsure about whether we could actually do it.

We went into partnership and opened Sh! in April 1992. I worked in the shop full-time. At first we were so unsure of our own survival that we only rented the shop on a week-by-week basis. We started the shop with six hundred pounds, and it has been in debt only once, when we bought a company car. The shop has done incredibly well; we have a loyal clientele that travels, often vast distances, to shop with us. We are also fortunate in that we get a lot of media attention.

Our shop is different from sex-shop chains supposedly run by women and catering for women. Many of these are a front for actual sex shops that cater mainly to men and use front women as an advertising ploy. We now employ two staff members, and customer service and care is our number one concern. We have approximately three hundred female customers per month, with an even split between gay and heterosexual customers. Plans for the business include deciding whether we want to wholesale the products we manufacture: the dildos and harnesses, and the handcuffs, collars, and other bondage gear.

I believe to have a good sex life you need to learn to tune into your true erotic nature. Come out about what you are interested in without shame. Explore your fantasies, and have the courage to live them out. But most importantly, ask for what you want sexually.

Tips on Introducing Sex Toys into a Relationship

✳ Introduce a sex toy into a relationship either seriously—via a slight power game with bondage or other fantasies—or with humor. A note of caution, though: if you buy sex toys with a partner, be aware that in a breakup these can become the objects of a custody battle, so buy your own sexual products.

✳ Imagination is the key to good sex. I defy anyone not to enjoy at least bondage (with no discipline). It is a wonderful feeling to be strapped down and made love to, because you don't have to think about anything—just relax and enjoy the sensations.

∗ You can sharpen your sexual skills by playing fantasy games—"playing" is the key word. If you can successfully re-create a fantasy character, you can feel that you are having an affair with someone else through the character. I have done this in my own relationship, and it has been a lot of fun. Sex toys can give an added dimension to a fantasy game.

∗ Strap-on dildos for women are the best-selling sex toys at Sh! It is a very common fantasy for a woman to want to experience wearing a dildo and harness. For a woman to strap on a dildo can be the most embarrassing thing at first, and you might feel like an idiot. You don't want your partner to laugh at you! One way to get over this is to blindfold your partner and introduce it that way. This will help you get over your initial awkwardness.

Women Can Orgasm Without a Penis

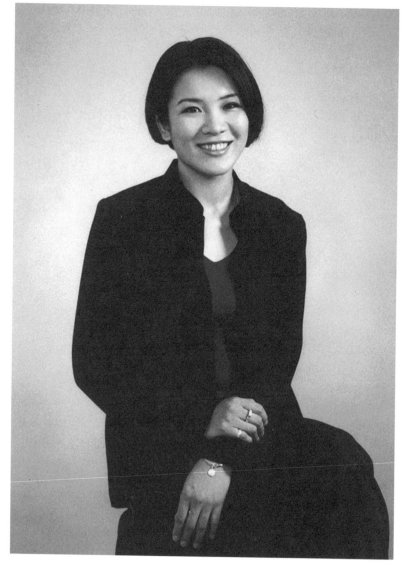

Minori Kitahara was born in Tokyo in 1970 and graduated from the school of pedagogy at a Japanese university. She now runs the Love Piece Club, a Tokyo adult shop and design/wholesale warehouse. Minori produces sex-educational material for women, including a recent groundbreaking booklet that shows women how to masturbate. While campaigning for a more open attitude toward sexuality in Japan, Minori is also leading the charge to produce nonviolent and less overtly macho pornography. In this, she is working with Japan's emerging feminist movement.

Minori has had a long interest in the sex industry. As a young girl she cleaned her grandmother's "love motel." Love motels are common throughout Japan, providing a place where couples can go to enjoy sexual privacy, as families often live together in relatively small apartments.

✳✳✳

When I first read Betty Dodson's book on masturbation, *Self Loving*, I was very moved. I said to myself, "I want to be a Japanese Betty Dodson." Now, my business is making and selling sex products for women. While we have many sex toys and videos in Japan, almost all of them show the fantasy of men with big penises conquering women. I hate this. Women need to have their own fantasies reflected, not just more of the same old porn.

Japan has twelve thousand adult shops, about four times the concentration of shops-to-people in Australia, and although nonviolent sexually explicit videos are illegal, explicit and savage sexual violence is quite acceptable on film and in print. Dildos and vibrators are also illegal, although if they have a "face" they are classified as "dolls" and so are acceptable. This has given rise to the distinctive Japanese vibrator, featuring a woman's or animal's face.

Prostitution is also illegal, but if a sex worker carries a whip she is safe, as she can masquerade as a bondage mistress. It goes without saying that Japan's sex industry and its sexual cultures are confusing.

I have designed and manufactured many innovative products, including a disposable dildo made from seaweed gelatin that dissolves in hot water after use. It is ideal for the busy couple who does not wish to leave "evidence" in their love motel or in their parents' living room.

I have also designed a remote control vibrator/dildo for women. The woman simply inserts a small, projecting section of the sex toy into herself and then positions the clit-tickling part, with the aid of snug underwear, before she goes out. While she's sitting at dinner, working out, on the dance floor, or attending church, the vibrator/dildo is activated at will by her partner via a small remote switch. The only problem arises when more than one woman in a room is wearing the sex toy!

For women to know what an orgasm is and what is pleasurable for them is very important. When we know this, we love our bodies more. Masturbation is the easiest way to learn this. We can then communicate our wishes to our partner and also be open to hearing what turns our partner on.

I don't remember when I started to masturbate, but since I was seven years old I've touched my genitals every night in bed before sleeping in order to feel comfortable. I remember my first orgasm— it was very sensational and happened when I was thirteen. One day I took a shower as usual, and the water pressure on my genitals gave me my first orgasm. Many of the women who come to my shop talk about having their first orgasm this way; often they can come during masturbation but not during sex.

It is not important to me to have an orgasm during sex, because for me sex is just a communication with people I love. In short, orgasm is not the purpose of sex. But many men are made very afraid by the fact that women can orgasm without a penis. And many women still feel guilty that they reach orgasm by masturbation. To me, selling vibrators means freeing women from the pressures of sex with men. I want to encourage women having orgasms—however it's done.

PART 10

Women with Women

When women are surveyed about their sexual fantasies, the fantasy of making love with another woman is always high on the list. The fantasy of breast touching breast, another soft body pressed against them, and feeling genitals with a sexual rhythm like their own seems to occupy many women's sexual imagination. The question is not why would a woman be attracted to another woman, but why wouldn't she? A woman can offer someone of her same sex a great deal in an intimate loving relationship. To women, another woman's particular emotional needs are not seen as peculiar or "other," but innately normal.

A woman knows how the female body works and has a firsthand insight into the nature of women's erotic pleasure. Women also have more sexual staying power, enjoying the ability to have multiple orgasms and to make love for hours on end. Put two of them in a bed together and you have dynamite.

When people are asked to place themselves on Alfred Kinsey's scale of one to ten, in which each end represents either absolute heterosexuality or absolute homosexuality, few people see themselves positioned immovably at either end. Most people recognize that there is ambiguity about their sexuality and that given the right time, place, or circumstance, an experience of loving someone of the same sex is quite possible. However, a gender difference exists here. Overwhelmingly more women than men admit to being open to the possibility of loving another person of their own sex.

Many women are naturally bisexual, but feel constrained by societal mores in the expression of that sexuality. For others, suddenly feeling sexually attracted to or falling in love with another woman comes out of the blue and can be a life-changing experience. Lesbianism—despite being the subject of endless straight erotic films—is still more taboo than male homosexuality, and surveys show that it is less socially acceptable. Every woman who decides to love another woman has to face a number of issues: negotiating a very different kind of sexuality, possibly "coming out" to friends and family, and learning to love and live in a very different manner.

Later in part 10, the contributors to this book who have had erotic interludes with other women offer their insights, experiences, and tips. One woman who has written on this is American sexuality author Susie Bright, and here she gives a practical and witty introduction to the concept of a woman picking up another woman.

Lesbians and Straight Men Have a Lot in Common

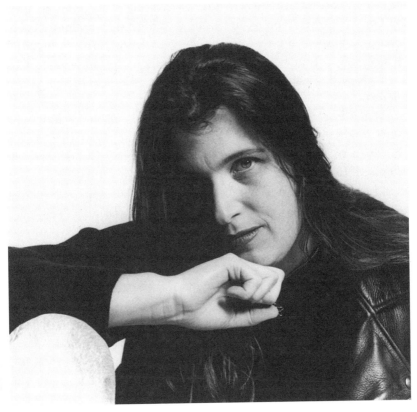

Jill Posener

Susie Bright is known as an editor, notorious sexual activist, advocate of sexual liberation, and performer. She is the author of Susie Bright's Sexual Reality, Susie Bright's Lesbian Sex World, Sexwise, *and her best-seller,* The Sexual State of the Union. *She is editor of the* Herotica *series of books and of the yearly anthologies* Best American Erotica.

Susie cofounded On Our Backs *and served as editor of the magazine for six years. In 1981 she began working at Good Vibrations, San Francisco's one-of-a-kind vibrator and sex-toy shop, where she created the first progressive feminist erotic video library. She lives in San Francisco and has a seven-year-old daughter.*

The following essay is extracted from Susie Bright's article, "How to Make Love to a Woman: Hands-On Advice from a Woman Who Does" (originally printed in Esquire *magazine).*

✳✳✳

As long as I've been searching for promises in the back of popular magazines, I've been drawn to that captivating title "How to Pick Up Girls." I'm sure you recall the ad. In addition to the untoppable come-on, it showed an average-looking bachelor carnally engulfed by a blonde, a brunette, and a redhead. His little smirk was calculated to lead us all to speculate on what his magnificent secret might be.

When I became old enough to pick up girls on my own—without a single guidebook to assist me—I thought about that cheesy Don Juan and whether I had acquired for free the wisdom his book promised for $19.95. Sometimes, during nights on the town, I would catch men staring at me and my latest girlfriend, their looks a combination of envy, bewilderment, and titillation. Their eyes seemed to beg for an answer to the question, "How?"

Lesbians and straight men do have a lot in common. Both are hung up on girls. We vie for the same joy. It's only natural for each of us to wonder if the other is having more success at it. Lesbians are certainly outmaneuvered by straight men—in numbers, influence, and earning power. And, they have penises. But I often think that if I had one, I'd really know what to do with it. (And I don't mean cut it off.) Lesbians know female sexuality from both sides, and so we have an internal, almost incestuous intimacy with the subject. It gives us a wisdom that can't be measured.

But it can be shared.

Suppose, for example, that I wrote a book called *How to Pick Up Girls Using the Real-Live Dyke Method*, including informative chapters on the following subjects:

The Look

For most humans, attraction begins with seeing. Look at her. All over. Linger anywhere you like. When she notices (and she will if you're really looking), hold her eyes with yours—hold them close. Every second will feel like a minute. This is the essence of cruising, and it is the experience that virtual reality and phone sex will never replace. It is also the one moment of truth: you'll know then and there whether she wants you or not. If she does want you, she'll be thrilled by your look, because it says to her that she has your full attention.

If she doesn't want you, she'll complain to her friends about how you "objectified" and "degraded" her, but ignore all that crap. Calling a man a sexist interloper is just a trendy way of stating an old-fashioned sentiment: "He's not my type." When a dyke gets an unwanted ogling from another dyke, we don't use political pejoratives. We just say, "Over my dead body." Don't confuse looking with watching. "Girl-watchers" check out every passing femme; to look, as *Webster's* so gracefully defines it, is "to exercise the power of vision."

The Touch

Lesbians, too, have probing, yearning, insistent sex organs. We call them hands. And if you have not had the pleasure of taking a woman in your hands—your thumb parting her mouth, your fingers tracing her ears, your hand curled up inside her—you are missing some of the finer points of ecstasy. Use your hands like they're your tenderest parts. The sweetest confession I ever made to a man was this: "You use your hands like a dyke." Lesbians often say that making love to a woman feels right because "it's like touching yourself." It's a flimsy reason for choosing a partner, but a good general motto for any lover. Touch your lover the way you would touch yourself. It's about empathy, not road maps. Every part of her corresponds to a part of you.

The Surrender

Consensual rough stuff aside, the thought that emotionally mature women (meaning no nut cases) enjoy mean and nasty treatment is way outta line. Women are invariably turned on by men who can be tender—it's like watching a statue cry, very moving. A woman hopes she will see more of this, and so she perseveres. Most times she learns that he's only vulnerable three days out of the year, and it's not worth the other 362 to wait for the High Holy Days.

Personality-wise you either have that candor and softness to express or you don't, but sexually anyone can lie back once in a while. Not every girl wants to get in the saddle and grab the reins, but if you have the slightest inkling that your woman would like to run this fuck, say a silent prayer and let her do whatever she wants.

My book would offer all that and more. But remember this bit of final wisdom: picking up girls is the easiest part of love. When it comes to seduction, you can try a dozen successful techniques. It's holding onto affection and lust that remains unteachable. The beginning of love is only the promise of all that's to come—for boys and for girls. Remember, it all begins with a look, which is nothing more than a hope, and if I can seduce a straight girl with the strength of my curious green eyes, then you shouldn't have any problem at all.

❊❊❊

KIMBERLY O'SULLIVAN You haven't lived until you have loved another woman.

ANNIE SPRINKLE For any woman who wants to explore herself sexually with another woman, I suggest finding a woman who defines herself as a lesbian, or who has had other female lovers. Avoid going after a heterosexual woman, because there is a high possibility of rejection. I have seen women frustrated and hurt by this mistake.

SHELLY MARS Ask friends who are lesbians to set you up with someone; lesbian bars are not my first choice. The dating relationship itself is not that much different from a heterosexual one—while courting, you go out to dinner, get some wine, and go home. I think a massage is always the best way to break the ice, because it relaxes someone. It's sensual but nonthreatening, and you can carry on a conversation while doing it.

If you feel that there is chemistry, kiss the other person, and go from there. Foreplay is no different whether you are with a man or a woman. If you are a woman you have a woman's body, so you automatically know what feels good and therefore you have an advantage over men. If appropriate, you could use some sex toys; be sure to ask her if it feels good.

DIANE TORR I have a game I play that goes like this: I do something you want for a certain amount of time, such as massage your back, suck your toes, stroke your hair.

You do something I want for a certain amount of time, such as kiss me all over my body, paddle my buttocks, lick me behind the knees.

Then we switch again, and so on. This is *guaranteed* to break the ice and is also a lot of fun.

NORRIE MAY-WELBY My tip is to make sure you're the same species as she is. Any human is capable of sexually fulfilling any other. If you're used to playing fixed gender roles, it may be useful to let these go. If everyone's waiting for someone else to be "the man," nothing is gonna happen.

The first time I ended up in bed as a woman with another woman, I remembered that my lesbian friends complained about straight women who laid back and expected the lesbian to do all the work. I resolved I wasn't going to be like that, because I identified as being good in bed! So I did my fair share of giving and receiving and was flexible about who took what roles.

Be responsive to your partner. Don't be afraid to do things that you may never have done with a man. Allow yourself to receive pleasure as well as give it. Penetration may or may not be part of what you, or she, wants. Don't assume it is, and don't assume it isn't. There is no set of orgasm techniques. Every woman is different and may even change herself from moment to moment.

Let go of expectations and preconceptions. Be as present in the moment as possible, and be with what's actually happening, not what you think "should" be happening. Respect stated and unspoken boundaries. You both have a right to say "yes, there, more," or "no, not there," and to change your mind at any moment. Most of all, bring your sense of humor to bed with you, and let yourself laugh, cry, or moan as the mood takes you.

CAROL QUEEN Ask her what she likes, and do your best to give it to her! If she's not sure or can't say, do lots of things, and have her give you feedback about what she prefers. Or give her erotic stories or videos to read or watch and ask her to find the parts she likes and wants to try.

In general (though there are exceptions), women like body contact. Our entire skins can be erogenous zones, so try a lighter touch moving to a more forceful or stronger touch as arousal builds. You want a wet, not dry, clitoris, so have lubricant handy! Many women love clitoral stimulation along with vaginal or anal thrusting.

These physical tendencies say nothing of the emotional ones. Does she like to be aggressive or to be taken? Does she want sex within a context of love and commitment? Or does she like to be out on the prowl? Each woman is different, so anyone wanting to please a particular woman has to pay attention to her responses and expressed desires.

CLÉO DUBOIS I come from a predominantly heterosexual background. When I came out into the scene in the very early 1980s, it was the beginning of many self-discoveries. I explored some simple kinky activities with women—spanking and whipping, for instance. In the queer community that welcomed me, some women were interested in playing with me as a submissive.

With them, and also with some gay leathermen, I discovered the joys of getting vaginally fisted. What an incredible, ecstatic, transformative experience! Until then I had no idea this practice even existed! For me it created a link between big orgasmic space, profound emotional depth, and spiritual awakening. From there, I began to identify as bi-kinky, playing often with nonseparatist leatherdykes as well as nonseparatist gay leathermen. Now, I certainly feel comfortable identifying as bisexual, although I'm not as confident of my sexual talents with another woman as I'd like to be.

Aggressive leatherdykes are the ones, and I hope will continue to be the ones, who have initiated with me if they are interested in play. I haven't had much experience with or much desire to be the initiator with femme kinky lesbians. There isn't a quick fix for these issues; for sex between women to happen at least one of them has to have some aggressive desires, and then I can't be guaranteed that I'll get "done" back! The ideal would be that both of you want each other and are vying for top or aggressive space. You'll just have to take turns! It's hard for me sometimes when women flirt with me and then won't do anything about it. I realize that they want me to do them, but if I'm not too interested, it just won't work.

I wish that we had the simplicity and directness that gay men have when cruising: picking each other up and making things happen. I'm looking forward to reading others' stories in this book to find some tips on how to do that! Gay men are also great at communicating their needs. "Rub this way, no that way, more there, do this, do that." Women seem to find articulating their needs that way very hard.

My friend Annie Sprinkle has created a fabulous workshop on ecstatic yoni massage, involving all kinds of techniques for pussy arousal, as well as one on anal awakening to pleasure. I always recommend these for men and women whenever they're offered. If you get a chance to attend, go for it.

For women, being sexual often seems to involve something of the heart. Gay men are so clear about sex for its own sake. We women are so much more complex! In my work with couples I have been happy to help women with no real same-sex experiences. Again, it seems that the mixture of role-play and sensuality can open doors that have been kept locked, even when the fantasy has been there for a long time. That is a joy!

KAT SUNLOVE As a bisexual, I have always found women desirable. As an assertive woman, I have rarely had trouble expressing that desire. My first experience with a woman is perhaps illustrative. My lover at the time was a handsome black man who knew of my interest in women. We were entertaining Jane, a close friend of mine from college, for the weekend. She and I had teased each other sexually over the years and had virtually traded boyfriends in school, but we had never acted on our erotic thoughts for one another. When Kenneth confided to me his desire for my friend, it excited me so much that I decided to try to make something happen.

When Jane prepared for a shower, I asked if I might join her and wash her back. The electricity between us at that moment told me all I needed to know. Had her reaction not been so clear, I'm not

sure that we would have ended up in bed. A simple opening like that
is not as difficult as a full-fledged seduction, in which you're per-
suading a reluctant female to explore the unknown.

But just as with SM, following the energy is the safest way I
know to explore sexual territory. If you feel an erotic charge when
you look in a woman's eyes or touch her hand by accident, you
should feel fairly confident that, if she is at all self-aware, she too is
feeling the same thrill. Whether or not she would wish to act on the
impulse is the risky part. Be brave. Look at her with intent in your
eyes. Let her see your desire, and if desire answers back you will
probably know what to do next.

DOLORES FRENCH I think being really direct is important. You can
meet women at events or places where there are lesbians or bisexuals.
When you meet someone you are attracted to and interested in
experimenting with, let her know and be direct. If you don't have
the guts, you won't have the glory!

NINA HARTLEY First, educate yourself about the nature of female sexuality, anatomy, and biology. A woman is drawn to confidence: people
who are at home in their skin and can transmit that to her. A woman
is drawn to people who are comfortable with touching: learn to
receive and give massage. Learn to kiss and pet. Learn to love cats
(if you don't already). Develop control over your own desire and
arousal. Be patient in bringing her up to your level. Don't be a user.

Learn to cook a couple of things: breakfast and a late-night
snack. Show consideration. Learn to appreciate beauty and art.
Being able to dance helps get a woman in a receptive mood. Learning emotional literacy and being able to communicate effectively are
of tremendous assistance. To fulfill a woman, you must arouse her
desire, make her want to be naked with you. The above-mentioned
skills are most useful in this task.

It helps to choose a sex partner who already masturbates, who
knows her body and can tell you what pleases her. To fulfill a
woman takes willingness and the ability to tune into her, to honor
her desires, even when they don't mesh with yours. Try to the best
of your abilities to help her live out her fantasies without disre-
specting yourself in the process. If a woman feels safe, respected,
and beautiful, she will be the most wonderful partner you can
imagine.

NAN KINNEY To heterosexual women who want to explore their sexuality with other women I say, good sex is all about communication. Communicate your desires to your partner whether you're straight, gay, bi, or whatever. There's no one way to fulfill everyone. You have to find out what your potential partner wants by whatever method you're good at: romance, reading a book together, playfulness, pretend, dress-up, watching a movie together (any kind of movie, but a porn movie would be best). Do whatever you can to open communication, to get the talking or writing going.

If you don't have a potential partner, try a workshop or read a book. Kim Airs at Grand Opening, a women's sexuality shop in Boston, leads a very successful workshop for women who want to explore lesbianism. Or you can read something like *Virgin Territories* about first times for women. See what's on the shelves in your local bookshop.

Should you go to a lesbian bar? Not with your boyfriend, not if you want a real lesbian! But seriously, if you're comfortable in bars, try it. See how you feel in a lesbian bar. Notice the women you're attracted to. Make eye contact. See if they return the contact. Then start a conversation. Talk about anything—baseball, politics, traffic. Bring a book or magazine with you and mention an interesting article or author you're reading. Buy her a drink. Words of advice, though: don't ever seduce a drunk woman. I don't believe drunk women can make cognitive choices about having sex. But you can get her phone number and meet for dinner or lunch at another time.

If you're not comfortable in bars, try lesbian events such as a reading at your local bookshop, or a softball game, or a motorcycle convention! Or church. Do everything the same, minus the drinks. Just remember to be yourself and not somebody you're not. Don't put on some "lesbian" image. When you're comfortable with yourself you are at your most attractive to other people. Relax. And if it doesn't happen the first time, there's always tomorrow. And there's always the vibrator when you go home.

JO-ANNE BAKER Communication is the key. If you are interested in someone, telling them that you are attracted to them will either take the connection further or clearly show you there is no interest. Why spend days, weeks, or months worrying whether someone likes you? It is so liberating to be able to just say it! In the traditional male-female interaction, there is much game playing. Women are meant to wait until a man shows interest, phones, asks her out, then she's supposed to wait again for him to contact her, if at all. If you call a man you are considered too pushy, too easy, too strong. In relationships with a woman the power dynamic is more equal, unless same-sex couples rely on gender stereotyping by taking on traditional male-female roles.

KY Being with a man is more problematic than being with another woman!

RUTH OSTROW My only comment to anyone wanting to experiment is go for it!

PART 11

Celibacy

Asking about celibacy in the hypersexual twenty-first century is like asking someone their financial status, religion, or political leaning—it is not deemed a suitable topic for conversation. Many women feel ambivalent about celibacy—is it a choice, a curse, a failure, a period of closed-off meditation, or a new way to view the world? Some women feel constrained by its solitariness, others freed by it. The question seems to hinge on whether women feel it was chosen or externally imposed.

Many people are confused about whether celibacy means refraining from sexual activity at all, or only sexual activity with another, meaning that masturbation is okay. For this discussion, we have taken celibacy to mean being sexual with yourself, but not with another.

For many single people, going without sex for weeks, months, or even years is not uncommon, yet the perception persists that this represents some kind of sexual failure. Celibacy is frequently portrayed as the refuge of the desperate, dateless, old, and unappealing. But is celibacy chosen because of a lack of *available* sexual partners or a lack of *suitable* ones? Many women choose celibacy to break destructive sexual patterns from repeating themselves. Others choose celibacy when they are in a state of sexual change or development, and still others choose it when they do not want the distraction of a lover because they wish to focus on their own creative growth.

Celibacy is not related to age, yet there is a widely held belief that the older you become the less sex you have, so by the time you reach your sixties, seventies, or eighties celibacy is inevitable. For those celibate in their twenties or thirties this view can be very destructive; people might falsely believe that if they are not sexual during this time, they will never have sex again.

There seems to be a belief in our society that if you are in a relationship you should be having sex as often as possible. To be celibate but involved with someone is considered even worse than being single and celibate. In such a situation many people believe that there must be something "wrong" between the partners. While there may be sexual issues that need to be addressed, many couples go through periods of celibacy without the love and commitment between them suffering in any way. Many people in long-term successful partnerships find other ways to show intimacy rather than having sex. If both are content with this situation it must be accepted as a valuable way of loving.

Celibacy proved to be one of the most controversial issues I encountered in my discussions with this book's contributors, even for women working in the area of sexuality. Frequently, my asking about it elicited a surprised silence, embarrassment, or even defensiveness from women who were otherwise articulate and sexually confident.

ANNIE SPRINKLE Sometimes celibacy can be a really positive experience. I have talked to many women whose celibate phases have formed an important part of their sexual evolutions. I know some people make the commitment not to have sex for an entire year or for a month because they wish to devote that sex time and energy to a specific project or to heal from an ended relationship. I have even known people in long sexual relationships with one partner who decided that they were going to, within that relationship, take a year and not be sexual together. It can be like an intermission from the passion and drama. Then you come back together totally renewed and rekindled.

There is a fine line between healthy celibacy and sexual repression, so be careful. Try to be clear about why you are choosing celibacy, whether you are happy about it or not. If you are not, change it. You can try to repress your sexuality, but it is going to be there; it will never go away. You might be able to sublimate it temporarily, but the sleeping dragons will awake and you will have to deal with them.

I don't know anyone who is celibate who does not masturbate.

As far as I know, everyone on the planet masturbates—as Dr. Joce-lyn Elders says, 90 percent of all people masturbate, and the other 10 percent lie about it.

ELIZABETH BURTON I think celibacy can be a positive thing because it allows time for yourself that can be spent getting to know who you are. There have been times when I rushed into going to bed with someone just for the sake of sex and felt sad and unfulfilled after-wards; I felt I had let myself down. If you are not in a fulfilling rela-tionship then you are either celibate or in and out of relationships. I don't want to be in and out of relationships—I would rather wait until the right person comes along.

LINDA MONTANO Celibacy can be a wonderful prayer.

CORA EMENS There might be a time for celibacy in everybody's life. Even though I never thought it would happen to me, since I absolutely enjoy sex, it did. Why? Because it did not feel right to have sex. There was no real longing for sharing since I was so busy getting to know myself on a spiritual plane. That was very impor-tant to me at the time, so I basically declared myself a "virgin" again, thus reclaiming full responsibility over my sexuality and my body. What I did from that point on was totally up to me.

During my spiritual quest, I definitely found something to work with and to work for. It is as if I understood my purpose in life. And that was the end of my celibacy! I am still very happy with myself and happy that I took the time to reflect on myself instead of indulging in the ever more meaningless pursuit of sex. Instead of renouncing my virginity, however, I announced my femininity.

Now I have a life partner, and we both enjoy a free and sexually open lifestyle with a nice mixture of meaningful and meaningless sex (!), and we are helping to liberate others through the media. I believe celibacy can be a good thing to experience, but we must understand that it comes for all persons in their own time. We can never force "morality" on people—in the end they will behave how and with whom they choose no matter what.

JWALA This is something I don't know much about. I have always wanted lovers and have had them in my life. The longest I have gone without a lover in my adult life is five weeks and the second longest is four weeks. Both times I had finished a relationship and was in a mourning process. When I finished mourning I met someone new to be sexual with. I express myself sensually and kinesthetically, so lovemaking and love affairs have been important for me.

KUTIRA True celibacy is not a denial or suppression of sexual energy. It is when one chooses to focus or channel sexual energy in nonsexual ways into life itself. There are times in our lives when this can be a personal love affair with oneself and an important phase in becoming ready to be in a healthy, loving relationship.

DIANE TORR Celibacy can be a time when you see no opportunity for sexual fulfillment in your life. It could be self-imposed in that you are 100 percent focused on a project and don't want to be distracted in any way. It could also be a time when you want to figure some things out. In a positive way, I think of celibacy as akin to fasting. You're cleaning the slate so that you can have a chance to recuperate and center yourself and learn about your sexual needs by focusing inwards. However, can you still be considered celibate if you masturbate?

In my own experience, celibacy hasn't always been satisfying or self-imposed. I'm just coming out of a relationship where there was a sexual drought for a number of years. It feels great to be horny, and I know I can reasonably expect sexual fulfillment with my new partner. What a relief!

NORRIE mAY-WELBY I have never consciously chosen celibacy, and have often felt frustrated when experiencing long periods of abstinence. Sometimes I could see that those periods were a result of my raising my expectations through improving my own self-esteem and then finding that available suitors would not likely meet my new personal standards. I have also had long periods without relationships where I was radically exploring myself in ways that I may not have if I had worried about a partner's reactions.

I have tried to ease my frustration during celibate periods by making lists of what needs are met from a relationship, and then finding alternative means of meeting those needs. I try to maintain a healthy sexual relationship with myself and not completely depend on someone else to fulfill my sexual needs.

SHELLY MARS I had a period of over a year when I was celibate. I think celibacy is a very healing time, allowing you to go into yourself completely and fully. It's interesting when the sexual drive goes away and you are just with yourself and you become alright about it. I think you focus more on yourself when you are celibate.

If people are in a relationship and celibate, I would at first think they were having some problems they need to work out. However, as I get older, I realize relationships can be tailored to fit everyone's needs, and if a couple is happy to be celibate and don't care, why should I?

Carol Queen I have not actually been celibate by choice—that is, I have not made a conscious decision to refrain from sex with others, which is how I mainly understand the term. However, I have been celibate for periods of time (a year and longer) in my adult life, because I haven't had a partner and haven't chosen to look for another. Also, I have been celibate for stretches of a few months while with partners with whom I wasn't being sexual, usually because the relationship was somehow in disarray.

Sometimes this "nonconsensual celibacy" has actually been exactly what I needed; it has been a grounding force that brought me back to myself when I was too focused on someone else.

I have not undergone any great length of time in which I've refrained from masturbation, and I do not see that I would ever choose to do so. However, at different times I have more or less sexual energy, so sometimes I go for periods without masturbating—but never by design. It simply has to do with my energy levels.

Kimberly O'Sullivan I was always very relationship-dependent, starting my first long relationship, of six years, when I was only thirteen. In retrospect it was way too young. I subsequently spent my entire sexually active adult life, until recently, in relationships or being actively promiscuous between them. I had absolutely no idea what it was like to sleep alone or to not have a sexual partner.

When at forty-one I became abruptly single, and nonconsensually celibate, I raged in fury against the universe. I felt in a state of utter abandonment. I had no frame of reference to see myself as an independent, sexually whole, single woman. I spent the next twelve months doing sexual therapy and counseling, exploring my own sexuality, meditating, and going within to search for answers.

I wanted to reconstruct my life and was determined not to repeat the same old mistakes I had made. When I came to the realization that there was no way I could do this without being single and celibate, I came to see my sexual and emotional state as a gift, not a punishment.

I now look at my year of celibacy as the best thing that could have happened to me sexually and emotionally. When I started having (plenty of) sex again I realized that something deep had shifted. I felt free of the desperate compulsion to be coupled—and my fear of aloneness had disappeared.

RUTH OSTROW I have had long periods of time without a partner, but I have never considered myself celibate, because I have had such fabulous fun making love to myself! In fact, some of my best orgasms ever have been at my own hand.

ROSIE KING In many cultures and societies, celibacy is very much valued. We are living in a particularly sexually obsessed era, where we practice "musterbation," (rather than masturbation, which is good for us). Musterbation is the belief that everyone must be having sex, when in fact every need met through sex can be met in other ways. You can express love and affection in nonsexual ways; you can find physical fun and pleasure in sports or other activities. You can experience a feeling of passion in work, community, or family. Anything that delights the senses will fulfill sensual needs, such as having a warm bath, playing beautiful music, applying lovely oils to your skin, massaging your feet, having a facial, or just brushing your hair.

To deal with skin hunger, you can find appropriate means of touch and affection by playing with animals or with children. Studies of dogs used in nursing homes and hospitals have shown that contact with pets seems to have a healing power, and the patient's health improves. All our sexual needs, including sexual release, can be met without sexual contact with another. Much worse than not having a sexual partner or not engaging in regular sex is having sex with someone you don't like.

Many people are involuntarily celibate, which feels very painful if it has been forced upon you. Alex Comfort, who wrote the *Joy of Sex*, said that old people give up sex for the same reasons people give up riding a bicycle—because they are not fit enough, they think it looks silly, or they don't have a bicycle. There are many women out there who don't have bicycles, so to speak. The Australian woman can expect, on average, up to ten years of widowhood, so we are left with an increasing population of older women without partners. Sexual fulfillment through solo sexual activity is something women need to explore, because you can have a terrific sex life on your own.

TUPPY OWENS I have used periods without shared sex to discover new sexual responses, but I hate the idea of not sharing a bed, if not every night, with someone I love and fancy. I also think that every day seems gray when there's not even one possibility that you might have a sexual encounter. I know there are Tantric practices that involve abstaining for months, with a fantastic outcome, but I can't see myself having the patience. I have always found that the more sex you have, the better it becomes.

AMANDA DWYER I think celibacy is unnatural. If celibacy is self-inflicted, I believe it would be because that person has no sex drive whatsoever or has taken an oath or vow for religious or spiritual purposes. If one finds oneself celibate because of circumstances within a relationship where one partner shows no interest, I think celibacy then becomes an imposed sentence.

Many of my personal clients have wives who are fully aware of their relationship and visitations with me and my establishment. Obviously, many people eventually make a decision about this. They come to a point where either they seek out a partner purely for sexual gratification, or they live in hope that things somehow will magically change within their personal relationship. I would see that decision as based on the level of commitment and trust that exists within the relationship. As long as commitment and trust are involved, there is always room for growth and the ability to overcome most negative things.

CLÉO DUBOIS First of all, I have to ask what we mean by *celibacy*. I once asked a female Episcopalian priest who came to me for a bondage and spanking session what she meant when she told me she was celibate. She said, "I do not have a vow, and of course I masturbate!" Does it mean being out of touch with your sexuality for a while, experiencing a lack of sexual drive because of loss, grief, depression, relationship difficulties, health problems, or hormonal life changes, even making a positive choice? I have a usually very sexually active woman friend who chose, after a relationship ended, to remain celibate for a year, except for masturbation, just to see how it would be. Obviously there's a big difference between choosing celibacy and either having no desire or wanting but not having a partner to have sex with.

During the mid-1970s I traveled to Guam, where there is a large American military base, and for six months I was isolated and without company. I didn't want to pick up sailors in bars, so I only had sex with my vibrator. That's how I discovered I was multiorgasmic! At another time in my life, I was very depressed, and although I was married and had a community of possible play partners, I didn't feel like having sex at all. It was only when I sorted out my issues through therapy that my sex drive came back.

So my experience of celibacy has been limited, but both positive and negative. I have read, and heard from women friends, that a period of celibacy can be empowering and centering, a time to find out how central your sexuality is to your identity.

Another friend was unpartnered for a while and was nonconsensually celibate. Having tired of her vibrator, she turned to the Internet and started to have lots of cybersex. In the process she tells me she found out a great deal about the nature of her desires and her fantasy life, which she subsequently brought into her real-life relationship when one eventually came along.

In my work with couples who are discovering the joys and challenges of BD/SM, it is not rare that the woman confides in me that the excitement of the new possibilities of role-playing brings sexual desire back into her life—and in a way where her whole body and mind become part of the arousal.

KAT SUNLOVE Well, there's celibacy and then there's orgasmic retention. Layne, my husband, and I practiced the latter in our early explorations of SM, deliberately allowing the Kundalini energy to build up to boiling point. It can be breathtaking when you are finally allowed to come. Orgasmic retention can make you want sexual contact so much that you are willing to do almost anything just for the mysterious sensation you crave. The senses are heightened by deprivation. That alone is an argument in favor of celibacy.

In later years, as we found ourselves less satisfied by routine SM play, Layne and I floundered around in our relationship, looking for an erotic combination that met both of our needs. We wanted to be sexual with one another because we were, and still are, very much in love. But the spectacular sexual experiences that we had enjoyed were not forthcoming with straight sex. We experimented with other people, as we always had in our very open relationship, and had some fun outside our primary partnership. But eventually we agreed that we would not work at sex, but rather would simply love one another and allow the sex to be there or not, without judging our relationship in a negative way if we chose not to be physical in our affection.

Currently, we are physically intimate very infrequently, either together or with others, but neither of us seems to mind. We love one another and know that we have enjoyed years and years of some of the best sex anyone could ever hope to have! And we fully expect we will again.

DEBORAH SUNDAHL Celibacy often signals a time of change in one's sexuality, one's desires or orientation or style. The old you is giving way to a new you, as yet unnamed and unformed, and so a transition period is necessary. And celibacy—refraining from regular sexual activity—emerges. Sometimes this involves a death of the libido altogether, and sometimes it is a choice to retain and acknowledge the erotic impulse, but not to satisfy it at all, or at least not in the usual ways: masturbation or partnered sex.

Celibacy is normally a temporary state, lasting from a few weeks to a few years. The best way to handle it is to acknowledge it as a time of change and to be gentle with yourself and your body. Listen to and explore whatever new impulses begin to emerge, however kinky or odd they seem at the time. In my case celibacy was an awakening to spirituality, and it required that I go into a state of seclusion so I could hear and give time to the new impulses awakening in me.

I believe celibacy is also necessary when one is breaking an addictive habit to sex or relationships, or, as Nik Douglas says in *Spiritual Sex*, if one has difficulty believing that sex is a sacred act. What replaces addictive behavior is the spiritual approach to life. What replaces a spiritual approach to life is addictive behavior. Celibacy is like a cleansing fast—it can be just as nourishing at times to go without food as it is to eat. When one takes the opportunity that celibacy offers to consolidate and examine one's erotic impulses and desires without the distractions and demands of a partner, one can emerge a clearer and more complete sexual being with renewed sexual energy.

DOLORES FRENCH I think it is very common for many couples to go through periods of not having sex, and I feel it is one of the last sexual secrets. In most cases, one of the people in the relationship has a problem and the other one doesn't. There are times when I don't feel like being sexual because of work, stress, illness, or excitement—and that is okay for me. There are times when I don't feel sexual, but these normally last a few hours as opposed to months. When I do things with my family that involve my nieces and nephews I find that I become nonsexual, and I can understand mothers feeling this way.

CANDIDA ROYALLE It can be very difficult when your lover is not interested in sex; it's difficult not to take it personally. Each one of us goes through times when we don't feel sexual. It does not mean that we do not love or desire our partner. If it goes on for a long time then there could be some problems that need to be addressed. It could be a time when you need to go into yourself and withdraw for a while. If you are a single person who does not want to have one-night stands, finding a good massage therapist is essential, because it is important to be touched and not to lose that connection with your body and your sensuality. You need to find a way to be sensual with yourself.

NINA HARTLEY I have had periods in my life with less sexual activity than others, but I have never been celibate, that is, voluntarily choosing to refrain from sexual activity with another person or myself. My job precludes me from being celibate, but when I'm away from my husband and wife (primarily when I'm on the road), I usually masturbate alone, even though opportunities for partner sex always present themselves.

If a person's decision to be celibate is a hysterical reaction to unresolved fears of sexuality, then it's merely a Band-Aid™ applied to a severed artery. If celibacy is deliberately used as a safe place from which to explore one's sexual issues, with intent to resolving them in order to live as a whole human being, then it's valuable. Celibacy in a relationship can only work with the agreement of all involved. One-sided celibacy will only lead to loss of intimacy, anger, resentment, and probable "adulterous" behavior in order to get basic needs met.

It's been my experience that celibate people are often on a spiritual trip, one that is alien to my sensibilities. I don't have anything against them, but I don't like to spend much time with them either. I find them concerned with subduing passion and desire, and I'm all about the freeing of those energies.

JOANI BLANK I respect people who are celibate, but it is not something I am attracted to, as I love being with people in a sexual way.

KY Celibacy offers a chance to make time for your own sexuality and to find out what you like and what sex does for you. I really like porn, so I would explore that. Don't put off satisfying yourself.

MINORI KITAHARA I used to be afraid both of being single and of being in a relationship. When I was single, I could not stand the loneliness. When I was in a relationship, I could not stand the restraints. Now I understand that whichever decision I make, I am what I am. The only difference between being single or in a relationship is the amount of room you have in the bed. I am not interested in marriage. In Japan, if women get married, they lose something important—freedom, pride, individuality. For many Japanese women, marriage means having no more dreams.

JO-ANNE BAKER I think all relationships go through times when one or both people don't feel like having sex. I just think of it as a normal part of life. I believe we all have different needs. Our need to be loved can be expressed and received in many forms. If we focus on sex as the only way to experience closeness and intimacy, we put a lot of pressure on ourselves and our partners.

There have been long periods in my life when I was single and chose to use my sexual energy in creative ways in the world. There was a two-year period when I didn't make love to anyone; I spent time exploring Taoist and Tantric breath and movement techniques, and I combined these with masturbation. I found it to be an invaluable time for experiencing great depths of inner pleasure. By the time I met someone I wanted to be with, our lovemaking became a new, exciting adventure that had a depth I had never experienced before.

PART 12

A Good Relationship

Everyone wants to know what makes a good relationship. We are not born with this knowledge; we learn it. Many people come from families that did not provide them with good role models for relationships. It is not uncommon for children to grow up never seeing their parents expressing love to each other or showing any displays of warmth, affection, or touch. Or the reverse is commonplace, and the home is a tense and hostile environment with emotionally absent parents. Often, one's concept of relationships comes from movies and television soap operas, which rarely mirror daily reality. The struggle of trying to balance financial stability and emotional security can cause much marital and relationship stress.

The 1960s shattered illusions about sexual roles, traditional marriage, and what makes a good relationship. As women became aware of a lack of personal and sexual satisfaction in their relationships, they developed new ideas about what they wanted. As women changed, so did the nature of their relationships. Women who were in unhappy marriages left their domestic situations, rather than "putting up and shutting up" as their mothers might have done in the past. Women wanted a successful relationship at home, as well as in the workforce; they realized they deserved to be treated in both arenas with dignity, respect, and equality.

Our expectations of relationships have never been higher and are in some ways unrealistic. People now look for a soulmate, lover, and friend in their partner, and if the relationship is not an exciting place, most of the time they vote with their feet and leave. Successful long-term relationships go through their ups and downs and are distinguished by the commitment of both parties to work through issues.

A "normal" relationship used to be a heterosexual marriage with
a dominant male partner who was the breadwinner, and a female partner who worked in the home and raised children. Today, such a stereotype hardly reflects reality; relationships encompass every combination of sexual expression, lifestyle, and domestic and financial relationship. Our era's social diversity gives us the freedom to have more satisfying relationships.

While the women profiled in this book are known for their work in the area of sexuality, they have all had to deal with the same love and trust issues common to intimate relationships. For some of them, their private lives have been enhanced by their public sex work and writings, while for others their private lives have had to carry the burden of their public notoriety. Their relationships and sexual identities cover every color of the erotic rainbow, and their collective wisdom about what makes a good relationship proves invaluable.

Some of these women are polygamous, some are monogamous, and others have been celibate for years. Some of them have been in longstanding marriages, others in multiple marriages or open ones. Some are heterosexual, others bisexual, others lesbians. Some refuse to be bound by any classification of their sexual identity. But there are some things they all agree on: a good relationship is characterized by trust, honesty, friendship, and a willingness to let both parties change and grow. And, of course, love and sexual compatibility!

ANNIE SPRINKLE To have a good relationship, you need to know yourself as well as possible: who you are and what you want. In my opinion, an ideal relationship is always based on being truthful, the freedom to be yourself, and the ability to share your feelings. I think you should always tell your lover if you are having sex with someone else, even if it might end your relationship, because it is important to base your relationship on truth. (Unless your lover says she or he doesn't want to know.) Always share the truth in a loving way. Make a commitment never to be mean to your beloved, even if you are really, really angry. Do yell and scream all you want, but don't cross the line into being mean. Always stay loving to your lover, and your lover will stay loving to you.

ELIZABETH BURTON Trust, similar interests, humor, and communication—these are essential to a good relationship.

CORA EMENS I am happy to be able to say that I have a good relationship with myself. I love myself, and more and more I forgive myself. Actually, I quite like myself as a person: I am smart, playful, sexy, creative, friendly, short-tempered, stubborn, and rebellious. I have learned to live with all my aspects instead of trying to get rid of certain parts of my character. Somehow it all seems to work together, just as a rose isn't a real rose without the thorns. You would not want to receive a rose from your lover without thorns, would you? So, since I love myself, why shouldn't my partner love me? Sound egotistical to you? I am happy to say that my partner and I have a good relationship. We both independently came to the same conclusion: only if you love yourself can you accept that someone else can love you, too. Only if you can embrace yourself with all of your flaws can you totally see through the rough bits of the "other." Then love becomes easy. We can still enjoy a good fight every now and then; after all, a sense of truth has the right to be defended! But we've learned how to fight without really hurting each other. The fight becomes part of the game—a game, a challenge, perhaps, but not a threat.

It is quite inspiring to get so passionately involved. We found great truths together this way. As long as you are willing to listen and respect your partner's viewpoint you cannot go wrong, you will love each other. As long as I or my partner can feel free to say whatever we think or desire, without the fear of being misunderstood, judged, or insulted, we have a good relationship. It doesn't always mean that you can fulfill your partner's wishes or that your partner expects you to. Allowing each other the freedom to experience whatever is necessary for one's personal growth is part of showing respect, having faith, and sharing.

My partner and I practice sharing with each other and with our kids, and in the meantime we improve the relationships we have with others. Some of them are close, others more anonymous. The relationships I have include myself, my lover, my daughters, my friends, the people I work with, and all the people whom I have met and will meet in the future, as well as relationships with nature and the spirit. I am on my way, but it will take some more practice!

JWALA Communication is the key to a good relationship. If you are holding back because you fear expressing yourself, it will affect how high and intense your ecstasy will be. The thing I have found to make my relationships work better is the ability to share and communicate and not withhold. I had a pattern of not saying anything when I was hurt or felt strange emotions, because I did not think I had the right to feel jealous. Now I express my feelings in words because it clears the air and I feel more intimate and present. Receiving clarification from the other person about what is going on with them also brings us closer. To find an art form or technique to create harmony is the goal. If there is a misunderstanding or projection, it needs to be cleared up as soon as possible.

KUTIRA When you are truly happy within yourself, that's when you can really meet another person who would be right for you. If you come out of neediness, if you need somebody, then you're in trouble, because such a relationship is doomed to fail. When you love yourself totally, and are happy with yourself totally, you can open yourself and love another. You come from a place of sustained fulfillment.

If I had met Raphael, my husband, twenty years earlier, we would not have made it. I had to first find that place of richness within. Twenty years ago I didn't have good communication skills, which are absolutely necessary for any relationship to thrive and grow.

There may be a time to experience your sexuality in an experimental way. But after a while your heart becomes more mature. Loving yourself creates a mature heart, which in turn creates trust and the ability to make and sustain a rock-bottom commitment. I finally found that I was running from intimacy. It was scary to commit my total being to somebody, all of who I am, the best and the worst; it was scary to become somebody who does not run away. Intimacy was the biggest step I had to take to allow myself to be vulnerable and to show truly who I am. But to be fully intimate you have to have the cornerstones of trust, integrity, commitment, and truth. Like a pyramid, without the cornerstones a relationship would fall down.

The other thing that seems to really work in our relationship is that we have boundaries. We are Tantra teachers; we are sensual with our friends, and that opens up many doors. But Raphael and I are a committed monogamous couple, and we totally honor that commitment. While I understand that each person and couple have their own choices to make about relationship boundaries, in our experience this works best for us. We practice sex magic, and that's for Raphael and me and our love. That gives our Tantric relationship a sacred space to grow and blossom to its fullest.

DIANE TORR Don't judge your partner maliciously. Love with a full heart. Give of yourself eagerly. Be attentive to ways in which you can honor the love you share, such as spending an erotic weekend away from your day-to-day life. Give time and space in your life to explore your interest in each other. Use strawberries dipped in chocolate liberally.

NORRIE MAY-WELBY Having been a partner to so many married people and others whose main partners think they're monogamous, I've had to look at how realistic my personal fantasy of a monogamous relationship was. Of course, as a sex-positive activist, I maintain that monogamy is an option that is no more right or wrong than other options, generally speaking. And I've looked hard at whether my goals in intimate personal relationships are harmful, harmless, pleasure-producing, or someone else's ideas that I've absorbed as my own without their really serving me at all.

I've concluded that, for me, emotional commitment is much more important than physical monogamy. I try to negotiate win-win rules where I can feel secure in a relationship while not restricting unnecessarily, or unrealistically, my partner's sexuality. Don't try to have someone else's relationship. Make your own. You are not your parents, nor are you someone in a movie or soap opera. Don't assume your partner has the same expectations you may bring to the relationship. Allow your relationship to be based on love and honesty, not on duty and covering up.

Be flexible and willing to negotiate and renegotiate the rules of your relationship, but make sure you respect your own bottom lines. Be willing to find what works for you, even if it may seem unusual or even "wrong" by someone else's standards. This is your relationship, not your mother's. Sometimes I have had to terminate relationships where my bottom lines were not being met. This doesn't mean my partners were at fault, merely that they were not meeting my needs. It is not ultimately their responsibility to meet my needs—it is mine.

Don't try to be everything for your partners, or insist that they depend only on you to meet their needs. It's only healthy for them to have friends and activities of their own, as it is for you. Allow each of you room to live and grow. A relationship should enhance your life, not replace it. Don't insist that this relationship be everything and forever. Be in the present with each other and yourself, not focused on tomorrow or yesterday.

Be gentle and play fair with each other. A relationship is not a competition to see whose will triumphs, or who is the most perfect wife/husband, girlfriend/boyfriend in the neighborhood. Or at least, it shouldn't be seen as a competition. The prize is not worth it.

Never stay in a relationship out of fear, particularly the fear of a lack of love. Don't just give your partner love. Make sure you give yourself love, too. The most important requirement for a good, loving relationship with a partner is having a good, loving relationship with yourself.

SHELLY MARS A good relationship takes communication—constantly asking and talking about how you feel, and then sharing this with your partner. It takes work and chemistry. Everybody has their secret demons inside; some people like to conquer and get somebody, and once they are conquered they have a fear of abandonment. So they have to leave the relationship first, or they have to see someone else secretly. If you know yourself, and you know why you do these things, it helps.

CAROL QUEEN Mutual attraction, the ability to communicate, and the desire and willingness to make the relationship work are the basic necessities, I think. Love, too, of course, though sometimes romantic love is a problem, particularly when it leads to unrealistic expectations and an unwillingness to deal with change. Romantic love is such a mainstay of many people's fantasies that it can be hard to focus on reality instead. Respect is as important as love, and really, the two aren't entirely separate.

Ideally, I think a relationship should be able to balance the heady and overwhelming energy of romantic love plus lust (which has been termed "limerance") with something more stable: a focus on commitment to whatever the participants have decided is important. People who have chosen to be together need to be able to call upon the magic of their togetherness and still deal with the real world: disagree without bitterness, negotiate expectations, support each other's individuality as well as supporting the relationship.

I think any number of committed people can have this sort of relationship as a goal: two, of course, but also three or more. With each added partner, finding the balance is more challenging, and negotiation and communication skills are more critical, but I have seen long-term more-than-twosomes work.

Other factors include compatible senses of humor and mutual interests (at least, be very interested in each other as people, not only as lovers) and compatible goals and standards around issues like work, money, offspring, monogamy, and so forth. Sexual compatibility, too, of course. A great relationship is one in which the participants like as well as love one another, are supportive as well as passionate.

KIMBERLY O'SULLIVAN Love is not enough; you need a whole lot more going for you to keep two people together. Don't lie, ever. Always think of the consequences of any action for yourself, your partner, and the relationship *before* the deed is done, not after.

Relationships are a two-way street. Always ask, "Am I getting as much as I am giving?" Don't be a rescuer, and don't be someone's mother. Make clear arrangements about relationship boundaries—what is emotionally okay with you, and what behavior crosses the boundary of acceptability. Communicate this clearly.

If you really love someone don't walk out when the going gets tough. Most importantly, when you fall in love don't lose your friends, your own identity, or your own life. Independence is essential to self-esteem.

RUTH OSTROW A good relationship requires two people willing to compromise over and over and over again—both with powerful senses of humor!

ROSIE KING It is very important to accept and understand gender differences in and out of the bedroom. Men and women are equal but definitely not the same. They have different communication styles and differences in sexual needs and responses.

Sex needs to be put in context—it is not the be-all and end-all of life. Sex in a relationship is like a glue and a lubricant; it is a glue because when sex is good it can bond the couple together, and it is a lubricant because when things are tough a loving sex life can smooth over the rough edges. I don't think sex is the most important part of a relationship. However, sexual difficulties can poison even the best relationship. Sexual difficulties should be dealt with as soon as possible, because they can be very toxic to the relationship.

We all need to learn each other's language of love; everyone learned a specific language of love in the home they grew up in. For some, touch might be the way love is expressed and experienced, for others it could be through words of love or gestures or spending time together. When two people who *speak* different languages meet they have to learn each other's language. Otherwise they are not going to be able to communicate. It is exactly the same with the language of love, and it is up to you to learn how to communicate love effectively. I need words of love, to be told that I am wonderful, lovely, and beautiful, and I need plenty of touch and affection. My husband, on the other hand, shows his affection by doing things for me and by spending time with me. This could be a recipe for disaster, except that we both have learned to be bilingual and to value the other's language of love. It is very easy to say, "You don't love me," but it may be that your partner is expressing love in a way that you simply don't understand or value.

I don't think everyone has to have a relationship. Obsession with having to be in a relationship, again, is what I call "musterbation." But I do think that long-term relationships of all sorts are very important in increasing our self-awareness. If you want romance and chemistry in your long-term relationship you really have to work hard. Love in a relationship is like a rare tropical plant: if you don't feed and nurture it, it will die. Lord Wagner said be a resident in your relationship, not a tourist. People think that they can be like absentee landlords, collecting rent from their relationships without maintaining the property. This is especially true of long-term romantic relationships. Because they are so intense, our partners are mirrors for us to look in to see who we are. Long-term relationships or marriages are also crucibles. A crucible is a high-pressure, high-temperature vessel. If you put a metal into a crucible and heat it up, the metal is transformed. I believe marriage does that. If you can stay the distance, it can transform you into a much better person.

TUPPY OWENS Everyone has different needs, but I would like to think that if people reversed their notion of a partner as someone they enjoy, own, or have to someone they give pleasure to, including allowing the freedom to have sex with others, then the whole world would be a happier place. Relationships are best when they are wild and free. You don't have to dwell on when they might end, but bear in mind that permanence is unusual and so not to be expected.

In Outsiders and in my own life it seems hard to strike the right balance between giving too much and not giving enough. But all you have to do is discuss with your partner whether you're getting enough.

AMANDA DWYER I have been married for many years to the same patient guy, whose constant support enables me to struggle through days when I think I never want to speak to another male again. We had both been through previous relationships, which for various reasons resulted in divorce and a number of children. We made a commitment to each other that we both wanted our relationship to work. We continue to take that commitment seriously. I guess it is still the main reason why we remain together today.

During this time I have also been involved in a dominant-submissive relationship with a guy who is my dominant partner. I believe you need to be able to live both dominant and submissive roles to be good at either position. For some reason I don't understand, I continue to be involved with my dominant partner. I often believe it gives me a real-life balance while running Salon Kitty's. I do know it is connected to my work.

Without our personal commitment, I doubt my husband would have persevered with my having this other relationship. Our commitment and trust keep holding us together. I believe they are the key elements to any successful relationship.

CLÉO DUBOIS There is no one simple answer to having a good relationship. What strikes me first as important is knowing yourself, knowing what you want, and being honest about it not only to your partner but to yourself. Ongoing communication is real work between partners. We now know that when we enter a relationship we bring to it not only our passion, our desire to love and to be loved, but also the luggage that our upbringings have burdened us with. In a sense, both partners bring to the relationship their own parents and the cultural norms and expectations they grew up with.

We need to sort out our issues so that we can know and understand what our needs are and have a chance to find fulfillment in some way. For me, a good relationship must be deeply rooted in heart space and love. As for sexual compatibility, two people can rarely fulfill all of each other's needs. We look for working compromises and agreements. It is possible to be an ethical "slut," and there are many ways to negotiate this, such as consensual, selective nonmonogamy. Parity and priorities are really important to pay attention to; this can be a delicate balancing act for both partners.

Exploring the boundaries of our sexuality, perhaps even across gender lines, having friends with whom we share some aspects of our sexuality—these things certainly enrich us and allow us to live our sexual lives to the fullest at least some of the time.

KAT SUNLOVE Communicate and forgive.

DEBORAH SUNDAHL Know thyself. Communicate thyself. Listen to what is being said and acknowledge it without attachment to what it may or may not mean to you.

DOLORES FRENCH Statistics show that, medically and emotionally, marriage is good for men, but divorce is good for women. Right before one of my marriages, I gave my attorney a small retainer for handling a future divorce settlement. He said, "This doesn't seem very optimistic." I said, "Get real. Marriage is the first step to divorce." A few years later my husband tried to retain him for a divorce. I'm glad I had planned ahead. I've had the same attorney through five marriages now. My most recent marriage has lasted eleven years and looks good for lasting quite a few more. Does practice really make perfect?

A friend of mine was furious when he came home unannounced from a business trip and found his girlfriend in bed with another guy. I told my friend, "If you want people to live up to your expectations, you usually have to provide them with the script, the props, and the cues." He had never specifically told her that he didn't want to find her in bed with another guy, and no arrangement had been made to avoid the offending scene. Instead of renegotiating, he chose to end their relationship.

Relationships are not sting operations. Often people believe that if they can manipulate their partners into an agreement, it's a done deal, no matter how unlikely it is that such an agreement can be kept.

CANDIDA ROYALLE A good relationship is based on communication and respect for your partner as well as taking responsibility for your own actions. Being compassionate to one another is important, but before you get to that place, I think it really helps to have a strong sense of who you are.

NAN KINNEY I have no clue about the requirements for a good relationship. My girlfriend will attest to this. But seriously, it's communication. The same as with sex, it all comes down to communication. (Taking out the garbage doesn't hurt either.) You cannot be afraid to express yourself. You have to be able to speak and to listen. You have to want to know how the other person's doing, to be attuned to each other's feelings. And you have to be assertive about those feelings, too; you cannot just hear that something is wrong and then not be willing to address it or do something about it. For example, my girlfriend was in a job that she hated, and she needed to talk about it every night. So I not only needed to listen to her feelings of unhappiness and fear and low self-esteem, but also try to come up with a way to work it out. To try to help her out of it. Relationships are not static; they're always changing, and you have to be okay with that. She finally left her job, but that was after many nights of sitting up late and her waking up in the middle of the night crying because she knew she had to leave the place that was making her crazy.

Respect is key. You have to respect the other person's individuality. Guard your lover's solitude, as Rilke wrote. So many lesbians just seem to become one, which often results in lesbian bed death. You need to keep your own interests, your own friends, your solitude or alone time, so you can continue to bring something to the relationship. I work out and run every morning for about an hour. That's when I can be alone and have my own thoughts. We try to make time for each other to have the apartment to herself. We have mutual friends and separate friends. It's not a big deal if one of us goes out and the other stays home and watches TV.

Your lover is a real live person, not just another part of you.

That takes work to realize and to act upon. I've had to work at it very hard. You have to be secure in yourself and do things that help you to feel secure. You have to like yourself, which is a problem for many women. You have to do things that make you feel good about yourself. That's why I run every day. I begin each day feeling good about myself.

NINA HARTLEY I know from personal experience it's not possible to have a truly good relationship without self-esteem and self-love. I've learned that one inflicts pain on others because one is feeling pain. If necessary, get therapy to resolve that primal pain and injury. If you do not love yourself, you can not permit anyone of quality to love you, and you will sabotage all relationships. Without self-respect, you will treat others badly, or will permit them to mistreat you while thinking you deserve it. Without self-esteem, you can only be servile toward others who show you kindness; you will be unable let their kindness or love heal you. You will be subservient to get their attention but unable to be submissive to your own heart.

JO-ANNE BAKER There are three main ingredients for having a good relationship.

Be affectionate with one another every day—cuddle before you go to sleep or when you wake up. Hold hands and touch one another in a nonsexual way. Often couples form a pattern when the only time they touch is when one of them wants sex. Problems arise when one of them does not want to have sex. Creating more intimacy in relationships starts with physical contact that is sensual and caring.

Say nice things to one another every day; expressing your appreciation and love for your partner is an essential ingredient. Initially it feels strange to say, "I really appreciate the care you took in doing that for me," "I love you," "You look sexy tonight," "I think you are wonderful/gorgeous/beautiful/handsome." After you start to compliment your partner you can see how he or she is able to relax and feel happy. It also encourages your partner to compliment you. For very busy people, leaving love messages on the answering machine or in notes is a creative way to remain connected.

Spend quality time together every week doing something you both enjoy. Many couples start to drift apart after a while because they have nothing in common. Taking up a new hobby or activity is a way of expanding your interests together. Spending time together in nature is a wonderful way to relax and unwind, as is getting dressed up and going somewhere special together.

Most of us fantasize about the ideal partner, but if we manifested a replica of what we thought we wanted, or a replica of ourselves, within a short period of time we would be arguing and discontented. I also believe that relationships are there for us to grow and are often a challenge because they cause us to look at ourselves, which can be painful. Remembering that we are doing the best we can is a way of being compassionate with one another when we are going through difficult times. Learning and putting into practice how to love another on a deep level is something that goes on until the day we die.

JOANI BLANK Many people get into talking about their relationship as a way to avoid talking about sex. You can pay lots of attention to your relationship, but the real problem might be a sexual one. Sex is always interactive. Anyone you are having sex with you are having a relationship with, even if it is only a one-night stand.

One book I would like to write is *No More Secret Affairs*, with the emphasis on the "secret," not the "affair." It would not be a book about how to avoid affairs, but a book about how to manage nonmonogamy. The particular form of nonmonogamy commonly practiced in the United States is where the couple is in a committed relationship, but one or both partners are having sex with someone else occasionally or on an ongoing basis. Statistics show that this occurs in two-thirds of relationships.

Typically what happens is that the man is caught, and he swears he will never do it again—which he may or may not—and they go on to live miserably ever after. Or at least *he* is miserable, because he likes to have affairs. The alternative is that the relationship ends. These are the only two options most people have. Most people don't consider the alternative that says, "Let's see how we can work this out in a way so that we can have sex with other people and it doesn't damage our relationship." I would like to interview couples who can successfully negotiate this for a reasonable length of time.

KY Communication and humor are the two most important things. Your partner should be your love star. I run a business with my partner of six years, and it could have finished us because we are so different, but we have instead negotiated a great personal-work split. In a relationship you have to acknowledge normal feelings like fear and insecurity.

MINORI KITAHARA Don't think you have to be nice to everybody. Love yourself.

Contact Information & Resources

Contacts

JO-ANNE BAKER For mail-order sexual products and to obtain information about individual sessions, contact The Pleasure Spot, PO Box 213, Woollahra, NSW 2025, Australia. Phone: +61(2) 9361-0433; fax: +61(2) 9331-6120; e-mail: pleaspot@ozemail.com.au; website: www.pleasurespot.com.au.

JOANI BLANK website: www.joaniblank.com.

CLÉO DU BOIS website: www.cleodubois.com.

CORA EMENS New Ancient Sex Academy, Boersstraat 30 sous, 1071 KZ Amsterdam, The Netherlands. Phone: +31(20) 664-4670; e-mail: corashai@hotmail.com; websites: www.c.e.emens@chello.nl, www.willemderidder.com, and www.come.to/coracoracora.

NINA HARTLEY website: www.nina.com.

JWALA For Jwala's workshops contact Good Vibrations in San Francisco, CA. Phone: (415) 974-8990; fax: (415) 974-8989; e-mail: goodvibe@well.com; website: www.goodvibes.com.

NAN KINNEY Fatale videos available through Good Vibrations in San Francisco, CA. Phone: (415) 974-8990; fax: (415) 974-8989; e-mail: goodvibe@well.com; website: www.goodvibes.com.

MINORI KITAHARA Love Piece Club, Tokyo, Japan. Phone: +81(3) 5226-9072; fax: +81(3) 5226-9093; e-mail: love@ummit.co.jp; website: www.ummit.co.jp/~love.

KUTIRA To receive newsletters and teaching schedules, or to order audio tapes or CDs, contact Kahua Hawaiian Institute, PO Box 1747, Makawao, HI 96768. Phone: (808) 572-6006; fax: (808) 572-0088; e-mail: kahua@OceanicTantra.com; website: www.OceanicTantra.com.

KY Sh!, 39 Coronet St., London, NI 6HD, UK. Phone: +44 (20) 7613-5458; fax: +44 (20) 7613-0020; website: www.sh-women-store.co.uk.

NORRIE MAY-WELBY website: www.cat.org.au/ultra/ultra1.html.

LINDA MONTANO For information about lectures, performance workshops, residencies, tours, and Art/Life Counseling, write to The Art/Life Institute, 185 Abeel St., Kingston, NY 12401. Phone: (914) 338-2813; website: www.rubylamb.com/lindamontano.html.

TUPPY OWENS For information about Outsiders, Sex Maniac's Ball, and the Sexual Freedom Coalition, contact Tuppy at PO Box 4ZB, London W1A 4ZB, UK. Fax: +44 (20) 7493-4479; e-mail: info@sfc.org.uk; website: www.sfc.org.uk. Donations welcome. *Planet Sex: The Handbook* costs $36.20 (checks to T. Owens).

CAROL QUEEN Carol's videos and books can be bought through Good Vibrations in San Francisco, CA. Phone: (415) 974-8990; fax: (415) 974-8989; e-mail: goodvibe@well.com; website: www.good-vibes.com.

CANDIDA ROYALLE website: www.royalle.com.

DEBORAH SUNDAHL Deborah's videos on female ejaculation are available through Good Vibrations in San Francisco, CA. Phone: (415) 974-8990; fax: (415) 974-8989; e-mail: goodvibe@well.com; website: www.goodvibes.com.

ANNIE SPRINKLE Annie's products can be ordered through Gates of Heck in New York, NY, phone: (718) 935-0227, and through Good Vibrations in San Francisco, CA, phone: (415) 974-8990; fax: (415) 974-8989; e-mail: goodvibe@well.com; website: www.goodvibes.com.

VERONICA VERA Miss Vera's Finishing School for Boys Who Want to Be Girls, PO Box 1331, Old Chelsea Station, New York, NY 10011. Phone: (212) 242-6449; e-mail: webhostess@missvera.com; website: www.missvera.com. To receive a copy of Veronica Vera's book, write to 85 Eighth Avenue, New York, NY 10011.

Books, Videos, and Multimedia

Women Sex-Performance Artists

Heidenry, John. *What Wild Ecstasy: The Rise and Fall of the Sexual Revolution.* New York: Simon & Schuster, 1997.

Jarrett, Lucinda. *Stripping in Time: A History of Erotic Dancing.* New York: HarperCollins, 1997.

Sprinkle, Annie. Herstory of Porn: Reel to Real. Video, 1998. Available through Good Vibrations in San Francisco, CA. Phone: (415) 974-8990; fax: (415) 974-8989; e-mail: goodvibe@well.com; www.goodvibes.com.

Sprinkle, Annie. *Post-Porn Modernist: My Twenty-Five Years as a Multimedia Whore.* San Francisco: Cleis Press, 1998.

Sprinkle, Annie with Beatty, Maria. *The Sluts and Goddess Video Workshop, Or How to Be a Sex Goddess in 101 Easy Steps.* Video, 1992. Available through Good Vibrations in San Francisco, CA. Phone: (415) 974-8990; fax (415) 974-8989; e-mail: goodvibe@well.com; website: www.goodvibes.com.

Spiritual Sexuality

Anand, Margo. *The Art of Sexual Magic: How to Use Sexual Energy to Transform Your Life.* New York: Putnam Publishing Group, 1996.

Connop, Cynthia (director). Sacred Sex. Video, Tantric Arts Pty Ltd., 1995. Available through Good Vibrations in San Francisco, CA. Phone: (415) 974-8990; fax (415) 974-8989; e-mail: goodvibe@well.com; website: www.goodvibes.com

Douglas, Nik. *Spiritual Sex: Secrets of Tantra from the Ice Age to the New Millennium.* New York: Pocket Books, 1997.

Jwala, *Sacred Sex: Ecstatic Techniques for Empowering Relationships.* San Francisco: Mandala, 1993.

Gender-Bending

Bornstein, Kate. *My Gender Workbook*. New York: Routledge, 1998.

Califia, Pat. *Sex Changes: The Politics of Transgenderism*. San Francisco: Cleis Press, 1997.

Dinshaw, Carolyn and Halperian, David M. (editors). *GLQ: A Journal of Lesbian and Gay Studies*, vol. 4, no. 4, 1998.

Feinberg, Leslie. *Stone Butch Blues*. New York: Firebrand Books, 1993.

Vera, Veronica. *Miss Vera's Finishing School for Boys Who Want to Be Girls: Tips, Tales, and Teaching from the Dean of the World's First Cross-Dressing Academy*. New York: Doubleday, 1997.

Women Scribes and Educators

Matthews, Jill Julius (editor). *Sex in Public: Australian Sexual Cultures*. Concord, MA: Paul & Company Publishers, 1997.

Mitchell, Susan. *Icons, Saints and Divas*. Sydney: HarperCollins, 1997.

O'Sullivan, Kimberly. *Magazines Kink*. Sydney: Wicked Women Publications, 1991.

Ostrow, Ruth. *Burning Urges*. Sydney: Pan Macmillan, 1997.

Ostrow, Ruth. *Hot and Sweaty*. Sydney: Pan Macmillan, 1997.

Queen, Carol. *Exhibitionism for the Shy*. San Francisco: Down There Press, 1995.

Queen, Carol. *Real Live Nude Girl: Chronicles of Sex-Positive Culture*. San Francisco: Cleis Press, 1997.

Tisdale, Sallie. *Talk Dirty to Me: An Intimate Philosophy of Sex*. New York: Anchor, 1994.

Wherrett, Richard (editor). *Mardi Gras!: True Stories from Lock Up to Frock Up*. Sydney: Viking Books, 1999.

Physical Challenges

239

Contact
Informa-
tion &
Resources

King, Rosie. *Good Loving, Great Sex: Finding Balance When Your Sex Drives Differ.* Sydney, Australia: Random House, 1997.

Kroll, Ken and Klein, Erica Levy. *Enabling Romance: A Guide to Love, Sex and Relationships for Disabled.* New York: Crown Publishers/Harmony Books, 1992.

Nestle, Joan. *A Fragile Union.* San Francisco: Cleis Press, 1998.

Owens, Tuppy. *The Outsiders Club: Practical Suggestions.* London: self-published, 1990.

Sex After 50. Video, 1991. Available through Good Vibrations in San Francisco, CA. Phone: (415) 974-8990; fax: (415) 974-8989; e-mail: goodvibe@well.com; website: www.goodvibes.com.

Domination and Submission

Brame, Gloria. *Different Loving: An Exploration of the World of Sexual Domination and Submission.* New York: Random House, 1993.

Califia, Pat and Campbell, Drew (editors). *Bitch Goddess: The Spiritual Path of the Dominant Woman.* San Francisco: Greenery Press, 1998.

Dubois, Cléo. *Fetish.* CD-ROM, Edge Interactive, 1996.

Wiseman, Jay. *S & M 101: A Realistic Introduction.* San Francisco: Greenery Press, 1996.

Oral Sex and Female Ejaculation

French, Dolores. *Working.* New York: E. P. Dutton, 1988.

Sundahl, Deborah. Videos on female ejaculation. Available through Good Vibrations in San Francisco, CA. Phone: (415) 974-8990; fax: (415) 974-8989; e-mail: goodvibe@well.com; website: www.goodvibes.com.

Winks, Cathy. *Good Vibrations Guide: The G-Spot.* San Francisco: Down There Press, 1998.

Film and Pornography

Hartley, Nina. Deep Inside. Video, 1993. Available through Good Vibrations in San Francisco, CA. Phone: (415) 974-8990; fax: (415) 974-8989; e-mail: goodvibe@well.com; website: www.good-vibes.com.

Rimmer, Robert (editor). *X-Rated Videotape Guides,* vols. 1, 2, and 3. Amherst, NY: Prometheus Books, 1986, 1991, 1993.

Stoller, Robert J. *Porn: Myths for the Twentieth Century.* New Haven, CT: Yale University Press, 1991.

Stoller, Robert J. and Levine, I. S. *Coming Attractions: The Making of an X-Rated Video.* New Haven, CT: Yale University Press, 1993.

Women's Sex Shops

Blank, Joani (editor). *First Person Sexual: Women and Men Write About Self-Pleasuring.* San Francisco: Down There Press, 1996.

Blank, Joani with Whidden, Ann. *Good Vibrations: The Complete Guide to Vibrators.* San Francisco: Down There Press, 2000.

Winks, Cathy and Semans, Anne. *The New Good Vibrations Guide to Sex.* San Francisco: Cleis Press, 1997.

Wiseman, Jay. *Sex Toy Tricks: More Than 125 Ways to Accessorize Good Sex.* San Francisco: Greenery Press, 1996.

Women with Women

Bright, Susie. *Sexwise.* San Francisco: Cleis Press, 1995.

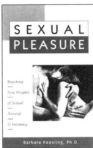
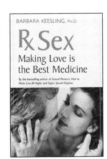

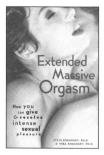
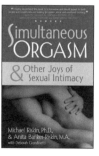

Other Hunter House books on SEXUALITY AND SENSUALITY

MAKING LOVE BETTER THAN EVER: Reaching New Heights of Passion and Pleasure After 40
by Barbara Keesling, Ph.D.

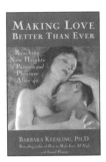

Great sex is not reserved for those under 40. With maturity comes the potential for a multi-faceted, soulful loving that draws from all we are to deepen our ties of intimacy and nurturing. That is the loving that sustains relationships into later years. In this book, Dr. Barbara Keesling shows couples how to reignite sexual feelings while reconnecting emotionally. She provides a series of relaxation, body-image, and caress exercises that demonstrate the power of touch to heighten sexual response and expand sexual potential; reduce anxiety and increase health and well-being; build self-esteem and improve body image; open the lines of communication; and promote playfulness, spontaneity, and a natural sense of joy.

208 pp. ... 14 b/w photos ... Paperback $13.95 ... Hardcover $24.95

SENSUAL SEX: Awakening Your Senses and Deepening the Passion in Your Relationship
by Beverly Engel, MFCC

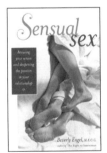

Life is a sensual experience that asks us to stop and listen, smell, taste, touch—and enjoy. *Sensual Sex* brings that dimension to lovemaking. It is about slow, sensuous, artful loving that feels good to both partners.

The one-of-a-kind "Reawakening Your Senses" program engages couples in a whole new level of physical exploration; "Deeper Love" offers an introduction to Tantric sex and sexual ecstasy; and "The Four Seasons of Sensuous Passion" discusses the stages of a long-term intimate relationship and sensual exercises that can strengthen each phase. Sensitively written and beautifully designed, this is a book to share, enjoy, and keep for a long time.

256 pp. ... Paperback $14.95

THE POCKET BOOK OF SEXUAL FANTASIES
by Richard Craze

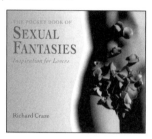

Our imagination knows no bounds when it comes to lust, passion, and sexual possibilities. But what sort of fantasies does your lover have? What can you share and what is best left unsaid?

This book explores why fantasies are important and how to get beyond inhibitions and act out your fantasies, how to set limits and say "stop" without undermining the erotic moment, and how to take turns. It guides readers through all the common genres of fantasy, including bondage, striptease, voyeurism, fetishism, toys, teasing, leather and lace, exhibitionism, and cross-dressing and touches on how fantasy can become an art form or a ritual.

96 pp. ... 64 color photos ... Paperback $10.95

THE POCKET BOOK OF FOREPLAY *by* Richard Craze

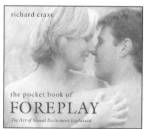

Foreplay isn't just a prelude to the "real thing"—it's an experience to be savored for itself. This book shows you how, with full-color pictures providing a guided tour of the joys of foreplay, from "Setting the Scene" to "Reaching the Limits."

Ever wanted to try foreplay at the office or fantasized about those sexy Tantric techniques? The full range of foreplay fun is here, adding an erotic new dimension to your lovemaking experience.

When a relationship falls into a routine that becomes boring, instead of looking for another lover to spice up your sex life try experimenting with foreplay to put sparkle and excitement back into your connection.

96 pp. ... 68 color photos ... Paperback $10.95

COMING in October 2001
THE POCKET BOOK OF SEX AND CHOCOLATE
by Richard Craze ... what more could a body want?

Prices subject to change without notice

Other Hunter House books on Relationships

INTELLECTUAL FOREPLAY: Questions for Lovers and Lovers-to-Be *by* Eve Eschner Hogan, M.A., with Steven Hogan

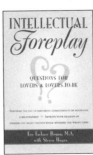

Do you want to find out whether a romantic partner is "the one"? Practice intellectual foreplay! This book of open-ended questions is arranged in thirty-four chapters ranging from *Romance and Sex* to *Values and Beliefs,* from *Sports and Hobbies* to *Money, Home, and Children.* It can help you get to know a partner—and yourself—in a deep, practical way, and improve your chances of finding the right partner while avoiding the wrong one.

Intellectual Foreplay includes guidelines for working with a partner's responses and steers you through a decision-making process, making it an exciting tool for discovery and growth.

288 pp. ... Paperback $13.95 ... as seen on MatchNet.com

DITCH THAT JERK: Dealing with Men Who Control and Hurt Women *by* Pamela Jayne, M.A., Foreword by Andrew R. Klein, Ph.D.

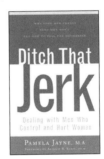

This is a women's guide to recognizing different kinds of abusive men— the potentially good, the definitely bad, and the utterly hopeless—and evaluating whether or not they will change. It is based on years of direct clinical experience with both victims and abusers and written for women who underestimate the dangers of an abusive relationship or overestimate their ability to change the man controlling or hurting them.

Neither weighed down with research nor weightless with airy promises, *Ditch That Jerk* is a gritty, honest, and experienced view of abusers and the effect they have on the women they victimize. Pamela Jayne shows how the minds of abusive men work, exposes the tricks and excuses they use to keep women in line, and even includes "jerk tests" to help you decide if you should walk. A potentially lifesaving book.

240 pages ... Paperback $14.95 ... Hardcover $24.95

To order books see last page or call (800) 266-5592

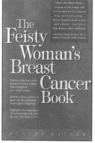
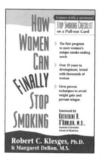

Other Hunter House books on
WOMEN'S HEALTH & SEXUALITY

WOMEN'S SEXUAL PASSAGES: Finding Pleasure and Intimacy at Every Stage of Life *by* Elizabeth Davis

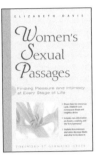

Davis unravels the mystery of how and why women's desire changes in the course of a lifetime under the influence of biological rhythms, hormones, and menstruation; pregnancy, birth, and child rearing; cultural attitudes, menopause, and aging.

Davis focuses on helping women to get in touch with their sexuality and also looks at the effects of stress, overwork, major life events, relationship upheaval, and sexual abuse. New chapters address sexual awakening, sex in the later years, and how hormonal changes at menopause can bring greater insight and assertiveness.

288 pages ... 8 illus ... Paperback $15.95

ONCE A MONTH: Understanding and Treating PMS
by Katharina Dalton, M.D. Revised 6th Edition

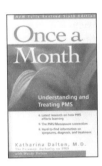

PMS has received the attention it deserves largely due to the work of Katharina Dalton. One-third of the material in this edition is new, from the latest research on how PMS affects learning to the PMS-menopause connection. Dr. Dalton also addresses the whole range of treatments, from self-care methods like the three-hourly starch diet and relaxation techniques to the newest medical options, including updated guidelines for progesterone therapy.

320 pages ... 55 illus. ... Paperback $15.95

ALSO AVAILABLE:

ANDROGEN DISORDERS IN WOMEN: The Most Neglected Hormone Problem *by* Theresa Cheung
One in ten women suffers from an imbalance of "male hormones," or androgens. This book describes the medical and emotional effects and outlines conventional and alternative treatments.

208 pages ... Paperback $13.95 ... Hardcover $23.95

ORDER FORM

10% DISCOUNT on orders of $50 or more —
20% DISCOUNT on orders of $150 or more —
30% DISCOUNT on orders of $500 or more —
On cost of books for fully prepaid orders

NAME _____

ADDRESS' _____

CITY/STATE _____ ZIP/POSTCODE _____

PHONE _____ COUNTRY (outside of U.S.) _____

TITLE	QTY	PRICE	TOTAL
Sex Tips & Tales... (paper)		@ $13.95	

Prices subject to change without notice

Please list other titles below:

_____		@ $ _____	
_____		@ $ _____	
_____		@ $ _____	
_____		@ $ _____	
_____		@ $ _____	
_____		@ $ _____	
_____		@ $ _____	
_____		@ $ _____	

Check here to receive our book catalog ☐   free

Shipping Costs

First book: $3.00 by bookpost, $4.50 by UPS, Priority Mail, or to ship outside the U.S.
Each additional book: $1.00
For rush orders and bulk shipments call us at (800) 266-5592

TOTAL _____
Less discount @ _____% (_____)
TOTAL COST OF BOOKS _____
Calif. residents add sales tax _____
Shipping & handling _____
TOTAL ENCLOSED _____
Please pay in U.S. funds only

☐ Check ☐ Money Order ☐ Visa ☐ MasterCard ☐ Discover

Card # _____ Exp. date _____

Signature _____

Complete and mail to:

Hunter House Inc., Publishers

PO Box 2914, Alameda CA 94501-0914
Phone (510) 865-5282 Fax (510) 865-4295
Orders: (800) 266-5592 or www.hunterhouse.com
email: ordering@hunterhouse.com

SXT- 2/2001